Working wit
Attachmen
Difficulties
in Teenagers
Practical & Creative Approaches

CW01507528

Working with Attachment Difficulties in Teenagers

Practical & Creative Approaches

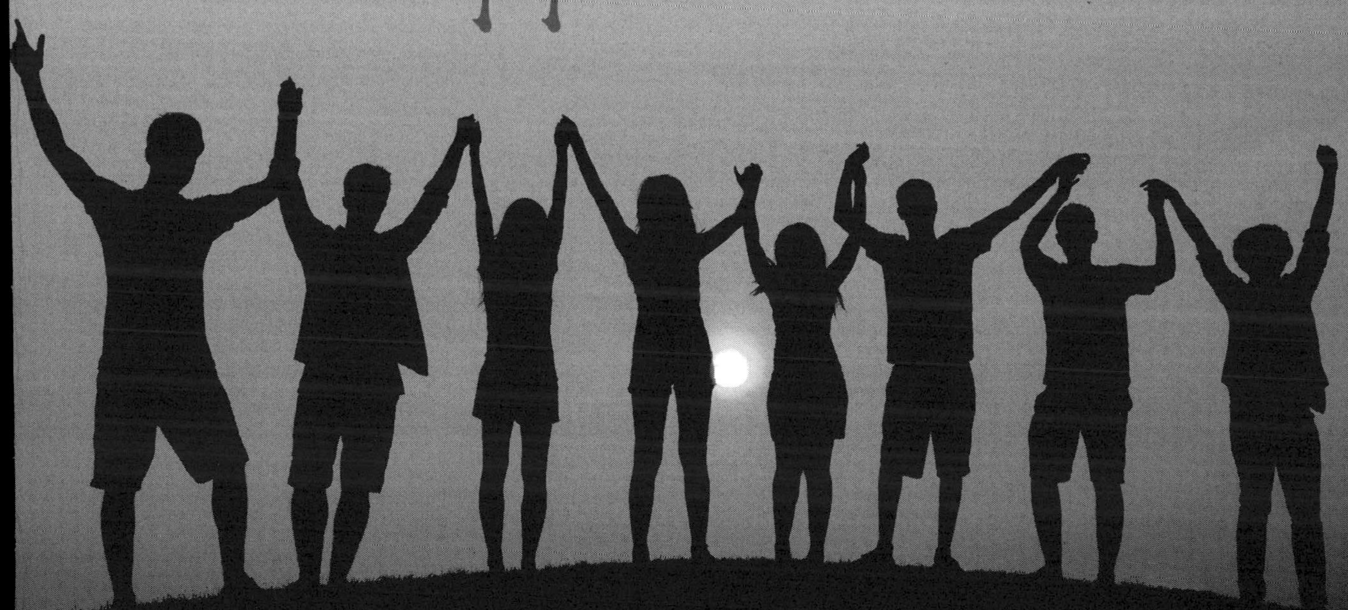

SUE JENNINGS

HINTON HOUSE Therapeutic Resources

HINTONHOUSE

Dedication
To Caroline Essame, MA,
art therapist and developmental play specialist,
a very special colleague and friend.

First published in 2019 by

Hinton House Publishers Ltd
T +44 (0)1280 822557 F +44 (0)1280 822338
E info@hintonpublishers.com

www.hintonpublishers.com

© 2019 Sue Jennings

The right of Sue Jennings to be identified as author of this Work has been asserted by her in accordance with sections 77 and 78 of the Copyright, Designs and Patents Act 1988.

All rights reserved. The whole of this work including texts and illustrations is protected by copyright. No part of it may be copied, altered, adapted or otherwise exploited in any way without express prior permission, except in accordance with the provisions of the Copyright, Designs and Patents Act 1988 or in order to photocopy or make duplicating masters of those pages so indicated, without alteration and including copyright notices, for the express purpose of instruction and examination. No parts of this work may otherwise be loaded, stored, manipulated, reproduced, or transmitted in any form or by any means, electronic or mechanical, including photocopying or storing it in any information, storage or retrieval system, without prior written permission from the publisher, on behalf of the copyright owner.

Warning: The doing of an unauthorised act in relation to a copyright work may result in both a civil claim for damages and criminal prosecution.

British Library Cataloguing in Publication Data
A CIP catalogue record for this book is available from the British Library.

ISBN 978 1 906531 39 3

Printed and bound in the United Kingdom

Contents

List of Activities & Photocopiable Resources

Part 1 Nurturing Experiences

Part 2 Projective Play & Internet Games

Part 3 Drama: Roles, Scenes & Solutions

Part 4 Integrated Themes: Weaving the Threads

Worksheets

Story Sheets

Acknowledgements

Thank you to all the NDP students and practitioners in the United Kingdom, Romania and Malaysia. You have worked tirelessly to develop important playful attachment work with children, teenagers and adults.

I appreciate the support and help of nieces, nephews, grandchildren and children of friends and relatives. You are so playful and creative!

As always thank you to Sarah Miles for being such a great publisher, colleague and friend.

Sue Jennings
Glastonbury, Somerset
Kuala Lumpur, Malaysia
Brasov, Romania
2019

About the Author

Sue Jennings was awarded the lifetime title 'Professor of Play' by the European Federation of Dramatherapy for her pioneering work in Dramatherapy and Neuro-Dramatic-Play (NDP). She is Honorary Professor at the University of Derby and Honorary Fellow at the University of Roehampton. Currently she is establishing international training in Neuro-Dramatic-Play, which emphasises the importance of early playfulness for attachment and the development of empathy and resilience. NDP is also important in addressing the effects of trauma and abuse. In addition, she is undertaking research into 'Newborn Play' with a focus on 'building bodies, building brains'.

Sue has written many books, a number of which have been translated into Greek, Korean, Russian, Swedish, Hebrew, Danish and Italian. Her doctoral research was carried out with the Temiar people in the Malaysian rain forest, where she lived with her three children, and which has influenced her understanding of 'playing for life'. She also trains carers in 'Creative Care', which is attachment-based creativity, to apply in work with older people and people with dementia. She was awarded a Churchill Fellowship for Arts and Older People in 2012/2013. She is currently editing a series on Early Years & Play for Hinton House Publishers.

www.neurodramaticplay.com
www.ndpltd.org
www.playanddramapartnership.org
www.suejennings.com
www.creativecareinternational.org

Contact: drsue@ndpltd.org

Introduction

This is book is about attachment and emphasises that attachment is a *playful* experience. It is a practical book that demonstrates how playful and creative techniques can enhance attachment and promote healthy relationships between parents and teenagers, and between teenagers and their peers.

The pioneering work of Bowlby and Ainsworth (1969) led the way in understanding attachment in relation to the lived world of the child, teenager and adult. Therapy had, until that time, focused on the spoken word and the fantasy lives of clients and patients. Indeed, it could be said that Freud's ideas about seduction within the family, often imposed on patients through the therapist's own interpretation, were often abusive. These projections from the therapist often locked clients into an unhealthy focus on their imaginings, rather than addressing the actual events that they had experienced. It also meant that patients and clients struggled with the veracity of their lives as they tried to make sense of their therapists' perspective. Just as Victorian parents were seen as 'right' and not to be challenged by children, similarly patients should not challenge the interpretations of the therapist. If they did so, this was usually called 'avoidant', or 'defensive', or 'resistant' – all favourite words that therapists have invented to keep themselves in controlling roles!

A prominent writer who has influenced my own ideas is Alice Miller who shocked society by pointing out that violence in society could usually be traced to violence in child-rearing. She has written extensively about the childhoods of tyrants and world leaders, such as Ceauşescu, trying to understand their early experiences. She also challenges the accepted views of the analytic movement, and points out that child abuse was a banned subject for many years, and that the therapists who propounded its veracity were hounded out of the 'movement' and labelled psychotic:

> The outlawing of the subject of child abuse in psychoanalytic circles has a long history, dating back to Freud's betrayal of the truth in 1897 (see *Thou Shalt Not Be Aware*, p.107). Because Freud could not bring himself to confront the truth about his own childhood, he made his students suppress the truth of child abuse wherever it raised its head. The consequences were far-reaching. Several generations of followers,

men and women, allowed themselves to be blinded to the truth as well. As a result, their patients seldom dared to question psychoanalysis's instrumentarium of power or its misleading interpretations.

Breaking Down the Wall of Silence,1997, p.4

Miller refers to it as the therapist's game of 'Blind Man's Bluff', the bottom line of which is: 'Whatever your parents did to you, you deserved. Our job is to show you your guilt.'

I have personal experience of this dynamic when I struggled for many years in psychoanalysis, several times a week. I was trying to understand my own teenage experience of violence and sexual abuse. I was told that it was something I had wished for in my fantasies – that this abuse had happened in reality was not considered important. My situation was compounded by the fact that my own children were suffering serious neglect by me as I struggled financially to pay for several sessions a week, and had to be absent from the house in the early morning.

I am certain that my single-minded pioneering of dramatherapy with an emphasis on theatre, especially Shakespeare, was directly influenced by my search for a form of therapy that made sense to me as well as others. Time and again I had found that theatre was both a solace as well as a discovery. Being able to find myself through not being myself! When I carried out research with the tribe in Malaysia, which included understanding shamanic practices, another piece of the jigsaw made sense. Through shamanism I began to understand 'entranced being'. Dramatherapy includes the capacity to experience a state of 'entranced being'.

The Entranced Experience

The entranced experience of another world is a means of healing. It is comparable to the specific trance experience that I describe in my field work with the Temiar people (Jennings, 1995).

> An entranced session through rhythm, dance, music and heightened sensory stimulation, within a cultural context, allows 'other world' experience.

This 'other world' experience is also referred to as an 'altered state of consciousness'. This can happen through the arts and without recourse to drugs and alcohol, and without prescription medication or shock treatment.

Teenagers long for escapes from the dreary and the tedious. They are living in bodies that cannot keep pace with their brains. They are marginalised and scapegoated and feel confused about their roles and responsibilities. They are told, 'Don't be childish'; and then, 'You are not old enough!' And they are targeted by the commercial world as a group of people who spend money and consume plenty.

Teenagers are, as their name suggests, 'inbetweeners': without traditional and cultural rituals in our western society (rites of passage), they are often disorientated about their lives and the world around them. Some may suffer from sensory processing difficulties that have never been properly diagnosed. When the world is overwhelming it is easier to tune-out.

Attachment & Teenagers

Many teenagers have not experienced 'good enough' attachment in their early lives, for a variety of reasons. They may have experienced a re-run of a parent's own adolescent experience, which means that traumatised adults may rear traumatised children. Wolynn (2016) refers to 'inherited family trauma'. He suggests that, for many people, the story does not necessarily lie with us, but in previous generations. Wolynn has been on a personal odyssey to find a self-cure, a journey triggered by an ocular migraine. His story is important and very informative in relation to our fears and anxieties and their origins. There are a host of reasons for attachment not to take place and since initial attachment takes place at the pre-verbal level, it is not usually helpful to offer verbal therapy.

It is difficult to talk about attachments without also talking about brains, and it is difficult to talk about brains without acknowledging the importance of neuro-science and a greater understanding of how our brains actually work.

There has been a revolution in understanding attachment with the developments in neuroscience and brain function. The orphanage crisis in Romania provided raw data on the importance of healthy attachments and demonstrated that the lines between nature and nurture are not clearly separated.

More about Brains

The theory of the Triune Brain (Maclean, 1985) helps us to understand developmental issues in children and teenagers regarding behaviour and learning processes. If early trauma or fears have not been resolved, then higher brain function may well be impaired.

The amygdala or 'reptilian brain' is the most primitive and oldest part of our brains. It reacts to danger but also signals when we need food, drink, shelter and safety. However, many teenagers 'at risk' have other fears contained in their amygdala, for example, as a result of growing up in a violent family.

The 'mammalian' part of the brain is part of the limbic system and is shared with other mammals. It is responsible for the growth of nurture and care.

The 'executive' brain, contained within the frontal lobes, is where we make decisions after weighing up the evidence, and where we reflect and consider the implications of what we are doing. Higher order thinking belongs to this part of the brain.

The reptilian, mammalian and executive brain are all useful when we are considering the development of teenagers and the level of drama, play and storytelling that would be appropriate.

Arts and the Brain

With the development of research in neuroscience it is possible to understand more and more the importance of play, the arts and stories for brain development.

Whereas the left hemisphere of the brain is concerned largely with numeracy, logic sequencing and facts, the right hemisphere is concerned with feelings, creativity, the arts and intuition. It is also responsible for 'the whole picture' whereas the left hemisphere is concerned with 'the bits'.

Generally speaking, Western education focusses on education for the left hemisphere more than the right. The arts are seen as 'wishy-washy' when compared with the scientific facts that are reasoned through logic! That side of the picture is slowly changing as researchers learn more and understand that the two hemispheres of the brain have to work together. For example, we form a hypothesis through a hunch or an intuition, and then use our logic to prove or disprove it. Nevertheless, when the school is under pressure to perform well in exams, it is commonplace for the art and drama classes to be cancelled and replaced with extra revision time.

Whereas early education concentrates on learning through play, and the freer the play the better, there needs to be a gradual balancing as the child gets older and becomes a teenager; it should never become out of balance and result in the left hemisphere dominating the right.

However, moving forward from the Triune Brain, and the right and left hemispheres, there is now newer research that demonstrates the influence of the arts and storytelling on the brain.

There are four main areas that illustrate the research:

1. Dopamine

The brain releases dopamine into the system in response to a pleasurable, emotional event. This is important because it helps us to remember the event more easily.
Therefore, we need to think about how our creative activity can be a 'pleasurable, emotional event'. Uninspired dramas, or stories that are read out like telephone directories will not engage anyone: they need to have timing and tone, vocal variation and suspense. They need to catch our attention.

2. Mirror Neurons

Mirror neurons respond when an action is performed and also do so when the same action is observed in others, so they 'mirror' the behaviour of the other person.
A recent discovery in neuroscience is the exciting knowledge of mirror neurons. They make a huge impact on the brain of the developing child in terms of the way adults behave as well as the 'role-modelling' for family life events and the sharing of stories and performances. We share the magic moments of a story often with a collective response, just like an audience in a theatre; at its simplest: 'He's behind you' or 'Oh no he didn't!' However, it is common for people in the audience to have both an individual and group response at the same time, whether it is comedy or tragedy.

3. Neural Coupling

A performance of a play activates parts of the brain that allows the listener to turn the story in to their own ideas and experience. Listeners' brain activity mirrors the speaker's brain activity with a delay (Gross et al, 2010).
Extensive research has shown that our neurons 'couple' with others during communication, and in particular during creative performances. Prophets and charismatic leaders have shown that we can be swayed by a 'show' that has emotional content as well as appealing to our here-and-now sensibility.

4. Cortex activity

When the brain processes facts there are two main areas that are activated. However, an enacted drama or well-told story can engage many area of the brain, including motor, sensory and frontal parts of the cortex.
The importance of drama, play and storytelling is shown by the fact that they involve several parts of the brain. The motor part is engaged through both our physical reactions as well as our gestures. We have sensory reactions such as tension,

pleasure, disgust, surprise. The frontal lobes are involved in problem solving, memory, impulse control and language, as well as other important functions.

The Importance of the Body

We have moved forward from the fantasy relationships promoted by the early psychoanalysts, to a deeper understanding of the physical body and how a brain is built.

Many of the teenagers with whom we work suffer from trauma (Jennings 2014, 2015; Lowenstein, 2002). And it may be that is the 'developmental trauma' recently described by Bessel Van Der Kolk (2015) in his excellent book *The Body Keeps the Score: Mind, brain and body in the transformation of trauma*. He reminds us that trauma is not just the major air crash or tsunami or road accident. He has identified what he calls 'Developmental Trauma', which occurs in children and teenagers who are systematically abused, neglected or rejected over time. These teenagers feel unable to communicate what has happened to them as they cannot put their feelings and experiences into words. This means that creative and playful techniques are ideal for trauma healing.

However Van der Kolk also discusses the importance of consistency in child rearing. He suggests that children learn very early to 'switch off' when they do not experience 'good enough' attachment, and that this being 'shut down' is not necessarily as a result of trauma, but is directly linked to their attachment experience.

Through carefully applied therapeutic play, and especially Neuro-Dramatic-Play, there is a chance to improve attachments and 're-run' early experiences in a more healthy and reciprocal fashion (Jennings, 2011). Creative play is easily adapted to teenagers and young adults in an age-appropriate way. Many teenagers would refuse to participate in activities that they deem childish or babyish. However, it I found it interesting to observe that the homeless teenagers and adults I worked with in Romania thrived on messy and rhythmic play. These were young people who had been grossly deprived in early childhood, had run away from orphanages and lived on the streets, often sleeping on the railway stations. They were desperate to smoke and wrapped bits of wood bark in newspaper to try and get a fix. Very physical, sensory and rhythmic play seemed to fulfil their need for sensory stimulus.

It is the body that suffers when there is inadequate attachment: the body is a primary means of learning, both before birth and from birth onwards (Jennings 1998). Bodies also need to feel safe and, just as the womb was a safe place, the embrace of a mother's arms is usually a safe place. However, the teenager who is rejected or abused does not feel that their body is in a safe place. Being 'held' gives us body boundaries in which we feel contained, and without those boundaries we are lost and disorientated. Many young people are watchful and wary as they do not feel safe, and their bodies feel unsafe. Container play with younger children (such as playing inside cardboard boxes) is one way of creating a safe space: however most teenagers would not accept this form of playing. We need to stretch our own imaginations and ponder how we can provide greater safety and feelings of trust. It is possible to feel safe in a role or character, by pretending to be someone else, and perhaps through dressing up. People mistake dressing up as a sign that teenagers are ready to do role-play, when for some it is the wearing of another layer that disguises their 'true' self. Obese young people may feel the same. I also provide rugs or blankets for teenagers to wrap up when relaxing or listening to stories.

Theoretical Models: Neuro-Dramatic-Play (NDP) & Embodiment-Projection-Role (EPR)

These are two developmental paradigms that chart early development and form the core of creative group work with children. Rather like the chains of DNA, NDP and EPR create curls and swirls in how we think about the creative play process and how we apply it with groups and individuals. Above all, the emphasis is on play and its essential contribution to the health of children and teenagers (Bruner *et al*, 1985; Sutton-Smith 2001; Brown, 2008).

The underlying theory and the individual and group application of NDP and EPR can be facilitated for improving attachment and social and emotional growth, particularly with teenagers who struggle with their communication and behaviour.

NDP and EPR are 'value free': they do not rely on a particular school of psychological theory or model of therapy. Being based on detailed observation, they can be integrated into any psychological model or therapeutic or educational practice. However it must be also stated that developments in Positive Psychology (Seligman, 2002) have continued to influence NDP and EPR, particularly in emphasising what children are able do, rather than their 'deficits' (Jennings, 2011).

Neuro-Dramatic-Play is characterised by 'sensory, rhythmic and dramatic play' and influences the growth of healthy attachments (Jennings, 2011). It occurs six months before and six months after the birth of the infant. It is a part of the Embodiment stage (birth to 13 months) and is responsible for the physical development of the senses and internal rhythms of the child. NDP also includes the dramatic playfulness between a mother and her newborn, in particular the phase during which they start to imitate each other's expressions. This reciprocal relationship establishes physical well-being, sensory play and creative expression.

Neuro-Dramatic-Play makes a vital impact on the growth of the brain and the body, and the development of attachment.

Embodiment-Projection-Role (EPR) is a developmental paradigm that uniquely follows the progression of dramatic play from birth to 7 years.

NDP and EPR chart the 'creative development' of children, which is the basis of the child being able to enter into their imagination. The early attachment between mother and infant has a strong 'dramatic' component through playfulness and 'role-reversal'. Even in pregnancy the mother is forming a dramatic relationship with her unborn child (Jennings 2011, 2014).

Competence in the NDP and EPR skills are essential for a child's healthy growth. These skills support the following:

- Reinforcement of the attachment between mother and infant
- Strengthening and further development of the imagination
- Building a child's resilience through 'ritual and risk'
- Role-play and dramatic play, which in turn create flexibility
- Development of the experience and skills to be part of the social world.

Embodiment-Projection-Role provides the markers of life changes that are developed through play and drama from one stage to the next.

Embodiment

'During the 'Embodiment' stage, we can see the way in which the child's early experiences are received through the body and the senses. The child develops security and trust (Erikson, 1965, 1995) through the early physical and playful attachment of NDP' (Jennings, 2011). However body-focused activities need to be adapted in an age-appropriate way. There are many drama games (see Appendix 1, 'Drama Games & Warm-Ups') that promote trust, security in space, body confidence, and coordination.

The body-focused activities in Parts 1 to 3 of this book are essential for the development of the 'body-self': we cannot have a body image until we have a body-self (Jennings, 1998). The teenager needs to be able to 'live' in his or her body, which grows from being a secure part of the mother's body.

Our early physical and bodily experience comes through our proximity to others, usually our mothers or carers, as we are rocked or stroked or cradled. Already the movement has taken on a quality of ritual/risk: on the one hand we experience the ritualised rocking movement, and on the other we are bounced up and down with glee. Ritual and Risk are the dual components of early physical play, where infants feel safely held and contained on the one hand, but contrastingly enjoy the thrill of the 'danger' (Jennings 1998, 2011). Teenagers with unresolved issues often indulge in extreme risk, dance with danger and get thrills through drugs and alcohol. All of these are physical activities and have a damaging effect on their bodies if indulged over time.

There are many drama games and sports that can help teenagers to develop confident bodies. Even though their physical experience maybe be distorted through abuse, domestic violence and neglect, it is still possible to change the outcome. However, if we do not understand the physical impact of trauma then we cannot find an appropriate remedy.

Some therapists may find it difficult to consider using Embodiment in their work because of traumatic experiences in their own past, or with the ever-present fear of misunderstood touch and possible litigation. It is very important that therapists explore their own physical history and reactions to touch. Just as intergenerational experience can be transmitted, therapists can also respond from their own childhood experience. This is certainly toxic for clients and impedes any potential for change. Therapists sometimes cannot bear what their clients tell them and retreat into safe formulas for treatment.

One solution is working in groups and group movement is very good for social development. Parents need to know that touch may be involved in creative workshops, and that teachers and therapists are always vigilant.

Simple games can include the following (see Appendix 1, 'Drama Games & Warm-Ups' for more ideas):

- simulated tennis
- simulated jousting
- touch tig
- slow-motion race
- walk tall, walk small

Projection

Some teenagers may feel more comfortable with projective exercises and they need to be 'fail-safe'. Teenagers, through trauma or unsatisfactory attachment, are lacking in self-esteem and confidence. Often they have been rubbished and put down and may experience exclusion, so as not to spoil SATS results.

However, for example, if teenagers are able to use large surfaces and broad pens they can practise art and craft skills. Similarly, working with collage, montage and clay (Souter-Anderson, 2015) can reassure and give enough freedom for teenagers to create. Lynne Souter-Anderson describes a teenage client who initially took an interest in bird pictures and then modelled a clay bird who 'wanted to fly away'. I described a parallel example in my story 'Tools have very talkative personalities' (Jennings, 2011), about a teenage boy who carved a parrot.

Many teenagers make their Projective play very sensory. They like to have big soft toys, multi-textured clothing, and very bright colours. They also enjoy hot chilli sauces!

As they build their confidence, teenagers will often start to experiment with different projective techniques: painting, clay, drawing, carpentry, sewing and knitting. There is an increased pleasure in going from 'mess to form', from chaos to order.

If we can understand their feelings about mess and chaos, we can allow the type of activities that encourage expression and transition.

Role

Usually, before 12 months of age, small infants engage in dramatic play with family members, playing 'peeka-boo', imitating and entertaining. This is a very important activity, because it is paving the way for empathy and resilience. Children who do not engage in dramatic play will struggle with the Role stage of development (that usually follows Embodiment and Projective stages), and will often adopt a 'fixed role' as they grow into their teens. Examples of fixed roles are 'loner', 'baddie', 'clown or entertainer' and 'poser'. As teenagers they have difficulties forming relationships, understanding empathy, and struggle with role flexibility, which is necessary for resilience to grow.

Van der Kolk writes a good deal about fear and teenagers' lack of trust. It is all connected with lack of appropriate attachment in early life. This theme is also developed in my book on anger management (Jennings, 2014) in which I suggest that underlying a lot of anger and even violence is fear. However fear is not something that most teenagers will admit to, so it is transformed into anger, self-harming and eating issues.

Teenagers (and adults too) will often live up to a role that is projected onto them by their families or friends. And many of them will play out the role, confirming expectations. Parents will say, 'But you always wanted to …', and so the young person finds it difficult to change direction. Parents can be very ambitious for their children, who feel forced into restrictive paths that they outgrow.

As Van der Kolk writes:

> As a culture we are trained to cut ourselves off from the truth of what we are feeling … Traumatized people are terrified to feel too deeply. They are afraid to experience their emotions, because emotions lead to loss of control. In contrast, theatre is about embodying emotions, giving voice to them, becoming rhythmically engaged, taking on and embodying different roles.
>
> *The Body Keeps the Score*, p. 335

If you are fragile about your own identity, it may be risky to play someone else! Carefully applied sensory work, movement and projective techniques will slowly build up the necessary internal strengths to then take on roles and characters in plays and stories. However the opposite can also be true, as there are also teenagers who can increase their coping and resilience through playing roles or characters who have greater strengths than themselves.

Dramatic stages for observation

A description of the development of dramatic interaction in stages can help us assess where a particular child may be located on a continuum of dramatic development.

The first stage on this continuum is naturally the pre-birth drama. We see role-reversal in the mother, who answers herself when talking to her baby. The baby, in turn, responds to the mother's voice and reacts to music, rhythm and touch. After birth there are seven further stages:

1. The 'as if' or the 'dramatic response' stage, echoing play and imitation, usually with mother or carer: the adult echoes the child, the child echoes the adult.
2. My body–our body. Physical 'whole-body' play with the adult: bouncing up and down together, flying, dancing, and so on.

3 Peep-Bo! The adult puts their hands on their face and then 'appears' again; the infant enjoys the repetition and the length of time to 'reappearance' can be slowly increased.

4 Role-reversal. The child talks to a special toy and then answers 'as if' they are the toy; this stage usually occurs in solitary play, as a relationship is acted out between the child and the toy.

5 Ordering and re-ordering. Soft toys or farm/zoo animals are assigned roles and lined up. They are often given voices, feelings, or characteristics of good/bad, or good/naughty.

6 Creating narratives. Whereas earlier play had traces of the elements of narrative, children are now putting things together into a true story structure. It may be on an epic scale, or a very simple conversation and outcome.

7 Improvisation and story. The child is able to spend an appreciable time in improvising an idea or scene. This leads to experimentation and choices and changes. It may then lead to a story based on the improvisation and shows an understanding of free flow and structure.

Development in dramatic role stages 1 to 3 is usually achieved by 6 months; stages 4 and 5 by 3 years; stages 6 and 7 by 6 years.

One can see that many teenagers will not have achieved these stages and will feel 'all over the place' when exploring roles and creating narratives. The techniques in this book provide a means to achieve the developmental stages of roles and narrative, without resorting to childish games.

NDP, EPR & Attachment in Practice

It would be easy to assume that, now we have a rationale, a progression and a range of techniques, we just go and activate the process. However, we need to reflect on the actual process of facilitating the group work with teenagers. It is not a question of designing a syllabus; rather it is important to provide the right context and environment to encourage creativity and spontaneity. What is needed for teenagers to flourish?

Teenagers who are 'out of rhythm', chaotic or in 'fixed' role need a secure structure with 'signposts' in order for their own creativity to develop as individuals and in collaboration with others, so facilitating the attachment process. Basic social skills within pairs, small and large groups, can foster decision-making, self- management, role skills, observation and alertness. Improvisation encourages flexibility and testing of ideas.

The philosophy behind this work is the empowering of children and teenagers, which means allowing them to develop at their own pace and in their own rhythm. Usually they regulate themselves in developmental sequences without having to be directed. However many teenagers who suffer developmental delay will often need to catch up through the NDP/EPR stages. Part of the task of the group facilitator is to have available materials that are age-appropriate.

Resources

Materials and an appropriate space are essential, so that teenagers can move around, sit comfortably in the floor, use props and dressing-up clothes, and make a noise!

Suggested equipment Recycled materials (as much as possible); newspapers and magazines, scraps of fabric; crayons, paints and brushes; glue, scissors, stapler; clay or Plasticine; simple dressing-up clothes, (wide variety of hats and caps, scarves, cloaks, shawls, belts and large pieces of fabric).

Contract

Every group needs to agree that there are basic ground rules, such as: no-one gets hurt, either physically or verbally; equipment is not broken or destroyed; everyone's work is respected, including art work or ideas that people contribute; everyone learns to listen to what others have to say and to contribute their own suggestions.

Warm-Ups

Exercises and games to focus physical energy, encourage cooperation, and develop mental strategies (see further examples in Appendix 2, 'Drama Games & Warm-Ups'). For example:

Freeze! When you call out 'freeze!', everyone stands still and listens to a new instruction. Also a great way to calm down group energy that may be getting out of hand!

Structure

A session has a beginning, middle and end (leading to closure); the beginning is the warm-up(s), introduction of a story or theme; the middle is the main focus of the action; the end is the cool-down, reflection, sharing and closure. One thing needs to lead to another and the sessions should not be a series of unrelated exercises.

Instructions and ground rules need to be precise and clear, as should the beginning and end of activities. Discussion and reflection about activities can be encouraged with questions such as: 'Has anyone thought about ...?'; 'How do the characters feel?'; 'Are there things the characters are not saying?

All of the activities can be modified for use with either older or younger teenagers where necessary. Some teenagers might refuse to participate in something they feel is 'childish', while others will do so with delight. You may also need to make minor adjustments if working with teenagers who have special needs or developmental delay.

Using this Book

This book is divided into four parts and each part focuses on a major developmental stage of attachment. In Part 1 there is a range of Embodiment ideas to build up the initial attachment relationship. In Part 2 there are ideas for developing Projective play and the beginnings of role-play, together with the use of voice. In Part 3 there are progressive improvisations, role-plays and story ideas. There are important role-plays using brief scenes from Shakespeare's plays. Part 4 is a shorter section that integrates several themes and structures once mastery has been achieved in simpler creative forms.

The appendices contain worksheets and stories, as well as more ideas for drama games that can be used warm-ups, or starter sessions.

Please note:

These are not therapy sessions. They are ideas that can be incorporated into therapy or teaching, as well as being appropriate for parents and carers. It is likely that children with attachment issues may well disclose abuse, current or past, and it is important that these disclosures are taken seriously and referred through the school or organisation's abuse policy.

Part 1
Nurturing Experiences

Teenagers can often be hard to reach when lack of 'good enough' attachment has made its mark on how they feel and behave.

This section consists of carefully chosen techniques that promote healthy attachment and enable children to re-experience attachment relationships that were neglected or avoided in the past. Many of the exercises are ones that are familiar to children and adults. They reinforce secure experience rather than causing insecurity by opening the door to too many new occurrences.

Each technique has a description, learning outcomes, activities and a rationale for attachment relevance.

Most exercises are relevant for children of all ages and both individuals and groups. Where there are variations, these are indicated at the beginning.

Activities 1 to 17

Activities 1 to 17 are based on Neuro-Dramatic-Play: sensory play, rhythmic play, dramatic play.

These stages mirror the attachment activity during the 6 months before birth and 6 months following birth. It is a period of intensely playful activity and the exercises have been chosen to replicate, as far as possible, the primary playful activity in graded sequences.

Please note there are additional ideas for messy play and activities in Appendix 3.

Activities 18 to 30

Activities 18 to 30 move forward into Embodiment Play (the first stage in the Embodiment-Projection-Role sequence), with a focus on whole body movement. The exercises develop coordination as well as spatial awareness and develop the capacity to say 'no' through the body.

Embodying different toys encourages the imagination and prepares for later role-play work.

1 Hand Massage 1

⊙ Individuals & groups

Resources

Appropriate hand cream or diluted essential oils, where possible allowing participants to choose.

Description

Care has to be taken with the choice of hand cream and essential oils are sometimes preferable. If possible allow group members to choose the perfume they prefer. 'Hand Massage' is the beginning of young people learning how to nurture themselves.

Learning Outcomes

- Learning to self-soothe
- Awareness of tension
- Sensory calming through touch
- Sensory calming through smell

Activities

- Explain to the individual or class the purpose of the exercise.
- If possible show illustrations or pictures of hand massage.
- Each person takes a few drops of hand cream or oil on their palm.
- Encourage them to rub their hands, back, front and fingers.

Attachment Relevance

Simple massage helps to replace lack of early nurture.

This page may be photocopied for instructional use only. *Working with Attachment Difficulties in Teenagers* © Sue Jennings 2019

2 Hand Massage 2

⊙ Individuals & groups

Resources

Appropriate hand cream or diluted essential oils, where possible allowing participants to choose.

Description

This hand massage is more complex and involves following a series of specific instructions.

Learning Outcomes

- Further encourages nurture
- Understanding variations in touch experience
- Increasing sensory integration
- Following a sequence of instructions

Activities

- Each person takes a few drops of oil or cream on their palm. Rub the hands together in circular motion.
- Massage the back of the hand by stroking from the finger tips towards the body.
- Using the thumb, massage each palm using a circular movement.
- Using the thumb and middle finger, massage around each wrist.

Attachment Relevance

Simple massage helps to replace lack of early nurture.

This page may be photocopied for instructional use only. *Working with Attachment Difficulties in Teenagers* © Sue Jennings 2019

3 Hand Massage 3

⊙ Individuals & groups

Resources

Appropriate hand cream or diluted essential oils, where possible allowing participants to choose.

Description

Being able to massage the hands of another person is a very big step in terms of trust and confidence. It is most likely to be effective as a one-to-one activity or in small groups of three or four people.

Learning Outcomes

- Being able to trust another person to touch appropriately
- Allowing oneself to receive nurture from another person
- Trusting the self to give appropriate care
- Following sequencing in a calm order

Activities

- Create partnership between a trusting pair (individuals work with the facilitator).
- Take it in turns to lead the massage.
- Remind people of the steps in the massage (see Activity 2): rubbing the palms, backs of hands from the fingertips, thumbs and wrists.
- Give sufficient time to change over.

Attachment Relevance

Establishing touch and trust between two people is a very big step. It may be that people need to self-nurture for some time before they can trust another person.

This page may be photocopied for instructional use only. *Working with Attachment Difficulties in Teenagers* © Sue Jennings 2019

alm Breathing 1

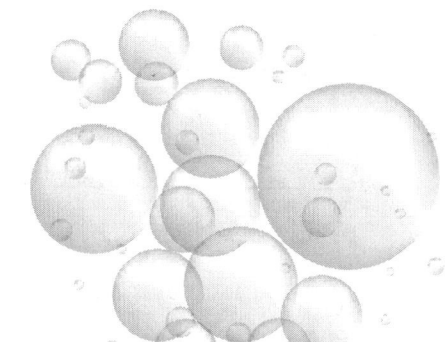

dividuals & groups

Resources

A quiet space with comfortable chairs, cushions/beanbags, or rugs on the floor.

Description

It is important to establish slow breathing patterns as a means of calming heightened emotion and anxiety. Early breathing patterns often become distorted in children through neglect or trauma.

Learning Outcomes

- Calm breathing enables the calming of emotion
- It encourages the slowing down of emotional energy
- It allows the individual to be in control of their breathing
- It increases their flexibility of communication

Activities

- Explain why calm breathing is important to reduce anxiety.
- Invite people to breathe in slowly through their nose and blow it out through their mouth.
- Make sure they are sitting comfortably with their back against the back of the chair.
- Repeat the breathing pattern six times.

Attachment Relevance

It is important for teenagers to learn how to re-establish calmness in their own bodies. This may have been disrupted through neglect or abuse.

This page may be photocopied for instructional use only. *Working with Attachment Difficulties in Teenagers* © Sue Jennings 2019

5 Calm Breathing 2

⦿ Individuals & groups

Resources

A quiet space with comfortable chairs, cushions/beanbags, or rugs on the floor.

Description

Regulating the breathing enables the individual to take control of their mood and feelings.

Learning Outcomes

- Encouraging relaxation
- Encouraging calm sleeping patterns
- Encouraging a variety of breathing functions
- Encouraging autonomy of breathing processes

Activities

- Encourage individuals to breathe in through their nose, pause and blow out through their mouth.
- Repeat this, but holding their breath for a count of 3 before blowing out.
- Experiment with increasing the pause time up to 5 before breathing out.
- Give a huge sigh to relax the shoulders.

Attachment Relevance

Developing breathing flexibility helps to replace panic breathing that is learnt at an early age, which often goes with hyperventilation.

This page may be photocopied for instructional use only. *Working with Attachment Difficulties in Teenagers* © Sue Jennings 2019

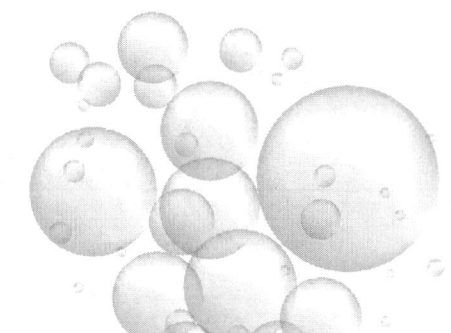

6 Calm Breathing 3

⦿ Individuals & groups

Resources

A quiet space with comfortable chairs, cushions/beanbags, or rugs on the floor.

Description

Lightly massaging the back of the neck and shoulders while breathing helps to reduce tension.

Learning Outcomes

- Understanding that the neck and shoulders are liable to express tension
- Enabling people to be proactive about tension
- Developing body image
- Encouraging greater autonomy

Activities

- Encourage people to lightly massage the back and the sides of their neck.
- Suggest that if they cross their arms to give themselves a hug they are able to massage their own shoulders.
- Suggest that if people breathe deeply during the neck and shoulder massage, it will increase its effectiveness.
- Finish by doing the exercise to the following count:
  - Count 2 while massaging the back and sides of the neck;
  - Count 3 and 4 while massaging the shoulders;
  - Count 5 and 6 while breathing deeply.

Attachment Relevance

The shoulders and neck are places where traumatised people usually feel most tension.

This page may be photocopied for instructional use only. *Working with Attachment Difficulties in Teenagers* © Sue Jennings 2019

7 Nurture through the Senses 1

◉ Individuals & groups

Resources

Choices of hot chocolate, hot milk and honey, fresh lemonade or other drinks that are not carbonated, or do not contain additives (see Appendix 2, 'Recipes: Nurturing Drinks', for ideas).

Description

Food and drink can be used to develop nurturing attachments.

Learning Outcomes

- Recognition of the role of food and drink in nurture
- Encouraging individuals to own their own preferences
- Avoiding, where possible, the use of additives in food
- Discouraging the use of artificial stimulants in drinks

Activities

- Explain to participants that food and drink can affect our mood.
- Encourage them to choose a drink (only one choice per person).
- While drinking, encourage participants to share memories.
- Suggest they measure their change of mood.

Attachment Relevance

Very specific drinks, particularly milk drinks, help to re-establish attachments and allow individuals to make associations with those drinks.

P This page may be photocopied for instructional use only. *Working with Attachment Difficulties in Teenagers* © Sue Jennings 2019

8 Nurture through the Senses 2

⦿ Individuals & small groups

Resources

Porridge, made in advance, or rice pudding.

Description

Experimenting with food that individuals find nurturing.

Learning Outcomes

- Re-educating peoples palates
- Encouraging the appreciation of food without additives
- Establishing the connection between food and mood
- Awareness of the physical and psychological ways food nurtures us

Activities

- Discuss early food experiences and likes and dislikes.
- Suggest that our moods can be affected by the foods that we eat.
- Suggest that porridge or rice pudding without additives are nurturing foods.
- Invite people to try porridge or rice pudding with, for example, raisins in it.
- Encourage their comments about food.

Attachment Relevance

Many teenagers will not have pleasant memories of their early food experiences. This exercise is the start of moving on from 'instant' food and an addiction to additives.

This page may be photocopied for instructional use only. *Working with Attachment Difficulties in Teenagers* © Sue Jennings 2019

9 Nurture through the Senses 3

⊙ Individuals & small groups

Resources

Ingredients for simple recipes (see Appendix 2, 'Recipes'); access to an oven, hob and cooking utensils.

Description

Involving individuals or small groups of teenagers in simple cooking, such as baking biscuits or making porridge, encourages both their experience of nurturing, as well as their self-esteem.

Learning Outcomes

- Developing new motor skills through cooking and mixing
- Encouraging accurate measurement of ingredients
- Building self-esteem by succeeding with 'no-fail' recipes
- Building sensory experience through smell, taste and touch

Activities

- Plan with the individual or group the recipe they would like to follow.
- Create enough time to see the process through until the end.
- Remember that cooking is an activity of creation and therefore boosts self-esteem.
- Share the food after completion.

Attachment Relevance

Many teenagers enjoy being involved in cooking, although of course this means having access to an oven and a cooking hob.

This page may be photocopied for instructional use only. *Working with Attachment Difficulties in Teenagers* © Sue Jennings 2019

10 Sensory Cooking 1

◉ Individuals & small groups

Resources

Choose a simple recipe that includes natural herbs and spices, including flavourings such as vanilla (see Appendix 2, 'Recipes') and prepare the ingredients; access to an oven, hob and cooking utensils.

Description

These techniques develop greater sensory awareness of textures, tastes and smells of food.

Learning Outcomes

- Increasing differentiation between the senses
- Awareness of different smells in cooking
- Awareness of different textures in cooking
- Encouraging the re-education of taste

Activities

- Place the ingredients on the table for individuals to smell and comment on.
- Encourage people to choose a herb, flavouring or spice they would like added to the food they are about to cook.
- Choose an appropriate recipe (see Appendix 2, 'Recipes') to cook together.
- Share the food at the end.

Attachment Relevance

Bearing in mind that early attachment focuses on the sensory experience with the mother or other carer, it is important to stimulate the ability to differentiate between the senses.

This page may be photocopied for instructional use only. *Working with Attachment Difficulties in Teenagers* © Sue Jennings 2019

11 Sensory Cooking 2

⊙ Individuals & small groups

Resources

Choose a recipe from the 'less sweet' category in Appendix 2, 'Recipes'. Prepare the ingredients and necessary utensils. Choose one that does not need cooking if there is no access to an oven or a hob.

Description

The recipes in Appendix 2 are to encourage not only healthier eating, but also to give teenagers the opportunity to be involved in the experience of nurturing themselves. The recipe chosen for this activity is one with a reduced sugar level.

Learning Outcomes

- Developing a taste for food unsweetened by sugar
- Changing the craving for sugars and non-artificial sweeteners
- Understanding the logic of alternative sweet foods such as dried and fresh fruit
- Encouraging self-worth to lead a healthier life style

Activities

- Discuss the different types of sugar and how certain sugars are harmful.
- Share some alternatives, such as raisins or chopped up fruit.
- Prepare the chosen recipe that involves alternative sweetening.
- Share the food and discuss.

Attachment Relevance

Attachment and sweetness in food are very connected. Addiction to sweet foods is very common in children and teenagers. This exercise involves a 'sweet experience' without the addition of harmful sugars.

This page may be photocopied for instructional use only. *Working with Attachment Difficulties in Teenagers* © Sue Jennings 2019

12 Sensory Cooking 3

⊙ Individuals & small groups

Resources

Choose a recipe from the 'sweet and spicy' section in Appendix 2, 'Recipes', and provide ingredients for participants to explore; access to a cooker hob and kitchen utensils.

Description

An exercise to encourage differentiation between spicy foods and sweet foods.

Learning Outcomes

- An appreciation of naturally grown herbs and spices
- An understanding of the role they play in cooking and medicine
- An ability to differentiate between the way that artificial additives (such as MSG) and natural ingredients (such as herbs) enhance food
- Pleasure in preparing and eating food

Activities

- Discuss the ingredients of the sweet and spicy recipe with the group.
- Support them while cooking the food, checking for any food preferences or allergies or avoidances.
- Create the time and place for sharing the sweet and spicy food.
- Encourage comments on the experience.

Attachment Relevance

The preparing and sharing of food encourages attachment between peers as well as teenagers and adults.

This page may be photocopied for instructional use only. *Working with Attachment Difficulties in Teenagers* © Sue Jennings 2019

13 Sensory Cooking 4

⊙ Individuals & small groups

Resources

Ingredients for one of the bread recipes in Appendix 2, 'Recipes: Sensory Food'; access to an oven and cooking utensils.

Description

This exercise is specifically about simple bread-making. It involves time and patience.

Learning Outcomes

- Encouraging the capacity to wait for results
- Understanding the different types of bread
- Understanding the role of bread in society
- Increasing self-esteem through successful creativity

Activities

- Discuss the role of bread and the different types eaten over the centuries.
- Consider the kinds of bread eaten in different cultures.
- Talk about the kind of bread you are about to make.
- Bake the bread and share with joy!

Attachment Relevance

The breaking and sharing of bread is a very primitive and human activity that connects people together. This is enhanced if the bread has also been made together.

P This page may be photocopied for instructional use only. *Working with Attachment Difficulties in Teenagers* © Sue Jennings 2019

14 Celebrations 1

⊙ Individuals & small groups

Resources

Choose a recipe from the 'celebratory' section in Appendix 2, 'Recipes', and prepare the ingredients; access to an oven, hob (depending on the recipe) and cooking utensils.

Description

The food is an important element in celebrating a birthday, a festival or a success. The emphasis here is on the significance of food that is homemade rather than shop-bought.

Learning Outcomes

- Acknowledgement of the importance of food in celebration
- The making and creating of celebratory foods
- The acknowledgement of the individual celebration
- The importance of food sharing

Activities:

- Try to share in advance with the group the choices for celebratory food.
- Show the ingredients and write them up on the board.
- Create the food and acknowledge who is celebrating.
- Share the food together.

Attachment Relevance

Many teenagers do not have affirmation of their individual celebrations and this acknowledgement helps to reaffirm their identity.

P This page may be photocopied for instructional use only. *Working with Attachment Difficulties in Teenagers* © Sue Jennings 2019

15 Celebrations 2

⊙ Individuals & small groups

Resources

Requires some preparation: at the end of the preceding session, ask individuals or group members to choose an activity and recipe (see Appendix 2, 'Recipes: Celebratory Food') that might celebrate an important event in their life (e.g., birthday, prize-giving). Prepare the resources in advance: you might need balloons, decorations, or even transport if individuals suggest a day out.

Description

It is important that each individual thinks of a celebratory activity and chooses a recipe that they would enjoy during their celebration.

Learning Outcomes

- Individual affirmation of identity
- Generosity of spirit between group members
- Allowing others to celebrate
- Increase in self-esteem and feelings of worth

Activities

- Ask individuals to discuss the meaning and importance of celebration.
- Talk about appropriate celebrations for individuals as well as groups.
- Explore ideas that the group would like to share.
- Make choices based on group's decision.

Attachment Relevance

When we celebrate important events with teenagers, it affirms their attachment experience, both as individuals and as a group.

This page may be photocopied for instructional use only. *Working with Attachment Difficulties in Teenagers* © Sue Jennings 2019

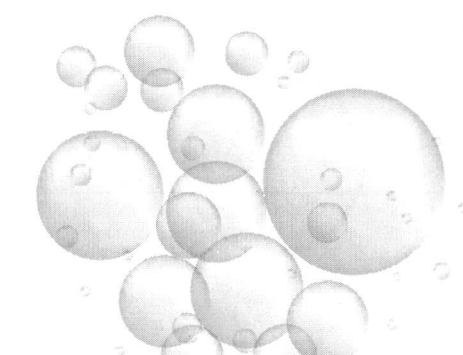

16 Sensory Play 1

⊙ Individuals & groups

Resources

Sufficient clay or Nuclay™ for each person to have the equivalent of a fistful; modelling board and wooden spatula per person, bowl of water.

Description

Messy play with teenagers, although important, has to be done with sensitivity. By using clay or Nuclay™, teenagers will usually accept this as a more adult activity.

Learning Outcomes

- Developing sensory awareness
- Being able to translate sensory awareness into model-making
- Satisfaction from being able to create an actual form
- Making connections between creation and self-esteem

Activities

- Encourage individuals to play with the clay: pounding, kneading it, rolling it, and so on.
- If the clay dries out, have a bowl of water ready to moisten it.
- Encourage group members to initially make shapes rather than objects.
- Create a final simple object, either a ball or a bowl.

Attachment Relevance

Working through messy play assists individuals to reconnect with primary experiences.

P This page may be photocopied for instructional use only. *Working with Attachment Difficulties in Teenagers* © Sue Jennings 2019

17 Sensory Play 2

⊙ Individuals & groups

Resources

Sufficient clay or Nuclay™ for each person to have the equivalent of a fistful; modelling board and wooden spatula per person, bowl of water, a garlic crusher, and or pasta maker.

Description

Developing modelling with the use of clay assists individuals to make connections by means of their own creativity and their art materials.

Learning Outcomes

- Developing the imagination
- Finding pleasure in artistic materials
- Developing further skills in modelling
- Creating a more complex shape

Activities

- Continue to 'work with' the clay.
- Encourage variety in shapes and forms.
- Suggest individuals choose the head of an animal or person to model.
- Experiment with dividing the clay into strands, using the garlic crusher or pasta maker.

Attachment Relevance

Creating forms with recognisable features slowly develops the concept of 'self and other'.

This page may be photocopied for instructional use only. *Working with Attachment Difficulties in Teenagers* © Sue Jennings 2019

18 Sensory Play 3

⊙ Individuals & groups

Resources

Sufficient clay or Nuclay™ for each person to have at least the equivalent of a fistful, with more clay available if desired; modelling board and wooden spatula per person, bowl of water; larger board for displaying landscape. Paints and paintbrushes, if desired.

Description

Creating a landscape with trees and animals helps people to 'manage' themselves in space.

Learning Outcomes

- Development of hand–eye coordination
- Awareness of the bigger picture
- Understanding spatial relationships
- Sharing the landscape (when working in groups)

Activities

- Decide on a landscape to be modelled, for example: countryside, seaside, village, and so on.
- Create individual trees, buildings and animals from the clay.
- Share (with other group members or the facilitator) the relationship between the objects.
- Allow the landscape to dry, possibly to paint later.

Attachment Relevance

By thinking about the relationship between modelled animals, trees and other landscape features, individuals are recreating their connections with others.

P This page may be photocopied for instructional use only. *Working with Attachment Difficulties in Teenagers* © Sue Jennings 2019

19 Drama Game 1

⦿ Groups

Resources

A large enough space for movement.

Description

Through drama games, teenagers are engaging in collaborative play and developing whole body movement and coordination.

Learning Outcomes

- Increasing confidence through the body
- Developing relationships with others
- Managing space
- Improving balance

Activities

- Everybody stands in a circle without touching.
- On a signal 'go', everybody has to run around the room and stops on a call of 'freeze'.
- Everyone makes a physical shape when called out, for example: tall, small, round, and so on.
- Intersperse running around the room between each body shape.

Attachment Relevance

Collaborative movement encourages physical and spatial relationships with others.

P This page may be photocopied for instructional use only. *Working with Attachment Difficulties in Teenagers* © Sue Jennings 2019

20 Drama Game 2

⦿ Groups

Resources

A large enough space for movement.

Description

Drama games are developed in more complex forms to encourage cooperation and non-verbal communication.

Learning Outcomes

- Development of 'body-self'
- Physical management of space
- Increasing awareness of others
- Fine tuning balance

Activities

- Stand in a circle and explain to the group that they are going to move towards the walls in different styles.
- Move towards the walls as if swimming.
- Move back to the circle as if horse riding.
- Add different movements, such as: walking the tight rope, wading through mud, slipping on ice, and so on.

Attachment Relevance

Physical confidence and coordination develops the equivalent of early 'body-self' management.

This page may be photocopied for instructional use only. *Working with Attachment Difficulties in Teenagers* © Sue Jennings 2019

21 Drama Game 3

⊙ Individuals & groups

Resources

A large enough space for movement.

Description

Developing a drama game in physical contact with a partner encourages trust and safe touch.

Learning Outcomes

- Awareness of bodily strength
- Experience of physical trust
- Working in collaboration
- Self-esteem and confidence

Activities

- Encourage group members to find a partner of approximately the same height. Individuals work with the facilitator.
- Ask the pairs to face each other and put their hands on their partner's shoulders.
- Ask them to try to push their partner across the room.
- Remind group members to use the strength in their legs, not only the strength in their arms.

Attachment Relevance

This exercise of 'safe struggle' encourages safe physical proximity and development of 'body-self'.

This page may be photocopied for instructional use only. *Working with Attachment Difficulties in Teenagers* © Sue Jennings 2019

22 Drama Game 4

⊙ Individuals & groups

Resources

A large enough space for movement.

Description

Continuing paired work and testing strength to build confidence and trust.

Learning Outcomes

- Increased awareness of 'body-self'
- Improvement of trust
- Development of 'grounding' experience
- Understanding of physical boundaries

Activities

- Find a partner of the same height. Individuals work with the facilitator.
- Hold the partner's hands and try and pull them across the room.
- Encourage the use of strength in the feet and legs.
- Repeat several times.

Attachment Relevance

This exercise of 'safe struggle' encourages safe physical proximity and development of 'body-self' awareness.

This page may be photocopied for instructional use only. *Working with Attachment Difficulties in Teenagers* © Sue Jennings 2019

23 Drama Game 5

⊙ Groups

Resources

A large enough space for movement; newspapers.

Description

By using newspapers to create 'islands', confidence and spatial awareness is increased.

Learning Outcomes

- Improving awareness of physical boundaries
- Coordination in space
- Developing increased flexibility of movement
- Sensitivity to materials

Activities

- Place several newspapers around the room, explaining they are islands.
- Everyone has to move from island to island.
- When 'freeze' is called, two people have to be on one island.
- Experiment with three people being on one island.

Attachment Relevance

Participants are collaborating physically and need to rely on each other for balance.

This page may be photocopied for instructional use only. *Working with Attachment Difficulties in Teenagers* © Sue Jennings 2019

24 Drama Game 6

⊙ Groups

Resources

A large enough space for movement; newspapers.

Description

Continuing the island theme, participants develop a greater awareness of working with others.

Learning Outcomes

- Increased awareness of the power of the imagination
- Relating to small groups as well as individuals
- Creating an idea of community
- Tolerance of others

Activities

- Invite participants to make groups of three or four.
- Suggest they use the newspapers to create their own island.
- Encourage them to create an island community.
- Share ideas and plans.

Attachment Relevance

By emphasising small group relationships, participants are slowly building up acceptance and trust.

This page may be photocopied for instructional use only. *Working with Attachment Difficulties in Teenagers* © Sue Jennings 2019

25 Drama Game 7

⊙ Individuals & groups

Resources

Scissors, newspapers, glue and A3 paper.

Description

Many participants are anxious about using their own words and by using words cut out of newspapers they begin to build their confidence.

Learning Outcomes

- Building literacy through newspaper words
- Encouraging group creativity
- Building ideas by sharing with group members
- Understanding of form and structure

Activities

- Invite people to form small groups and explain they are going to create a story.
- By cutting words out of newspapers they can make a collaborative story.
- Stick the words on the A3 paper.
- Share the stories together.

Attachment Relevance

Developmentally, group members are beginning to use language to create stories and structure.

This page may be photocopied for instructional use only. *Working with Attachment Difficulties in Teenagers* © Sue Jennings 2019

26 Drama Game 8

⊙ Individuals & groups

Resources

A large enough space for movement.

Description

By developing what is known as 'body percussion', rhythm can be stimulated in different body parts.

Learning Outcomes

- Experiencing rhythm through different limbs
- Awareness of movement and voice combined
- Experimenting with different sounds
- Developing the musical possibilities of the whole body

Activities

- Encourage group members to stand in a circle with space in-between them.
- Develop the body as a percussion instrument.
- Use the chest, the arms, the calves and the stomach to make different sounds.
- Make vocal sounds at the same time.

Attachment Relevance

Whole body awareness encourages internalised rhythms and creativity.

This page may be photocopied for instructional use only. *Working with Attachment Difficulties in Teenagers* © Sue Jennings 2019

27 Drama Game 9

⊙ Individuals & groups

Resources

A large enough space for movement.

Description

Group members are encouraged to work with a partner and to use each other's backs as drums. It is important to re-enforce the idea of the 'safe zone', from shoulders to waist.

Learning Outcomes

- Experiencing safe touch on the upper back
- Developing further rhythms in the rib cavity
- Sharing ideas with partner
- Tolerance of difference and similarity

Activities

- Explain that we can use each other's back as a percussive instrument, but only between the shoulders and waist.
- With a partner, one person chants, while the other beats a rhythm on their back.
- Vary the pace and pitch.
- Change around.

Attachment Relevance

This exercise establishes whole body awareness in an age-appropriate way that mirrors the early attachment experience between mothers and babies.

P This page may be photocopied for instructional use only. *Working with Attachment Difficulties in Teenagers* © Sue Jennings 2019

28 Drama Game 10

⊙ Individuals & groups

Resources

Scissors, glue, newspapers, A4 paper and coloured pens.

Description

Creating a poem develops the use of rhythm and form.

Learning Outcomes

- Improving self-esteem through creativity
- Encouraging rhythm with words
- Developing the use of metaphor
- Stimulating the expression of feelings through poems

Activities

- Discuss the idea of expressing feelings through poems.
- Write on the board as many 'feelings' words as the group can think of
- Suggest they can cut words out of newspapers to make their own poem.
- Decorate the poem and share.

Attachment Relevance

Encouragement of the expression of feelings enables individuals to move on in their emotional development.

This page may be photocopied for instructional use only. *Working with Attachment Difficulties in Teenagers* © Sue Jennings 2019

29 Drama Game 11

⊙ Groups

Resources

A selection of drums, if possible one for each participant.

Description

Having explored rhythm through poetry, the next exercise develops rhythm physically through responding to drumming and chanting.

Learning Outcomes

- Development of regular rhythmic play
- Internalising rhythms into one's sensory processing
- Linking rhythm to coordination
- Participating in rhythmic chanting

Activities

- Sit in a circle and take it in terms to invent a drum rhythm that others copy.
- Decide on the collective rhythm that everybody beats.
- Use the chant 'way-ay-yay' while beating the collective rhythm.
- Build up a piece of chanting and drumming that alternates individual and group rhythms.

Attachment Relevance

Many teenagers are out of rhythm as a result of early trauma and need to reinternalise a consistent rhythmic schema.

P This page may be photocopied for instructional use only. *Working with Attachment Difficulties in Teenagers* © Sue Jennings 2019

30 Drama Game 12

⊙ Groups

Resources

Supply of drums.

Description

It is important to connect rhythmic drumming with voice as well as physical movement.

Learning Outcomes

- Coordination of rhythmic movement
- Encouraging chanting with rhythmic movement
- Group coordination of rhythms
- Sensory integration of sound, voice and movement

Activities

- Explain to the group that they will be using not only rhythm and chanting, but also movement.
- In groups of three: one person can drum, while their partner moves and the third person chants.
- Encourage experimentation with movement and sound.
- Share contrasting activities.

Attachment Relevance

This complex exercise integrates the physical with the rhythmic and vocal, while incorporating the group's own ideas.

This page may be photocopied for instructional use only. *Working with Attachment Difficulties in Teenagers* © Sue Jennings 2019

Part 2
Projective Play & Internet Games

The activities in this section (31 to 60) contain many 'fail-safe' ideas as well as variations involving art and modelling. Internet games are also included.

Fail-safe techniques are important for building confidence and self-esteem: many teenagers feel they are no good at anything, having lacked the affirmation of self and its associated skills that is usually acquired during the early years. The 'Messy Monster' ideas are a means of allowing messy play at an age-appropriate level, although I have worked with teenagers and young adults who cannot wait to explore flour and water and finger paints!

Projective techniques with collage and paints allow young people to give form to feelings and embody their experiences through shapes and models. Their random, and sometimes chaotic, feelings about their situation can be expressed through different media. They are able to create images about their dwellings and environment. There are also exercises in this section to learn about our brains and to see how we can better understand our feelings through that knowledge. This is also important for self-esteem, since the word brain is a well-used in our everyday language, for example: 'no-brainer', 'brainy', 'brain-dead'.

This section closes with a variety of internet games and strategies. Some people may wish to start with these activities, since the internet is familiar territory for most teenagers and they feel at home with these techniques.

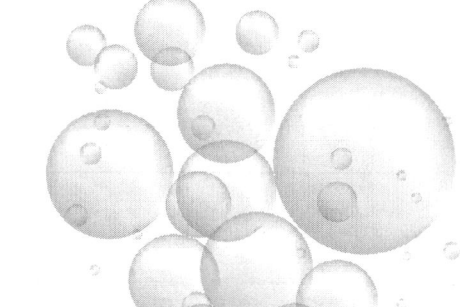

31 Messy Monsters 1

⊙ Individuals & groups

Resources

Thick paper (such as sugar paper), two contrasting colours of water-based paint, water, 2 plastic pots for each person, straws.

Description

This is a fail-safe exercise for participants to transform splashed paint into images.

Learning Outcomes

- Transforming random patterns of paint
- Increasing flexibility of thought and feeling
- Understanding that abstract paint patterns can be transformed into pictures
- Building confidence through creating images

Activities

- Put a small amount of paint into a plastic pot and dilute with water. Repeat with the second, contrasting, colour.
- Make two puddles with the contrasting colours on thick paper.
- Use a straw and take a deep breath and blow the paint in various directions.
- Continue blowing until the paint is disbursed.

Attachment Relevance

An acceptable means of messy play that creates art images.

This page may be photocopied for instructional use only. *Working with Attachment Difficulties in Teenagers* © Sue Jennings 2019

32 Messy Monsters 2

⊙ Individuals & groups

Resources

Thick paper (such as sugar paper), two contrasting colours of water-based paint, water, 2 plastic pots for each person, straws; a dishcloth each (e.g., fabric or kitchen roll).

Description

Following on from Activity 32, this is a fail-safe exercise for participants to transform splashed paint into images.

Learning Outcomes

- Increasing flexibility of thought and feeling
- Acknowledging unique art-making
- Understanding that abstract paint patterns can be transformed into pictures
- Building confidence through creating images

Activities

- Dilute the two contrasting colours of paint as in the previous exercise.
- Placing small puddles of paint on the paper, use the straw to blow a shape that looks like a head with spiky hair.
- Use cloth or kitchen roll to shape the head.
- Use the straw and the contrasting colour to create the features of a monster.

Attachment Relevance

Continuing creativity through messy play.

P This page may be photocopied for instructional use only. *Working with Attachment Difficulties in Teenagers* © Sue Jennings 2019

33 Houses 1

⊙ Individuals & groups

Resources

Old magazines and catalogues, scissors for each person, white glue and thick A4 paper.

Description

Use magazine images to recreate environments from the past.

Learning Outcomes

- Awareness of a previous life situation
- Communicating important factors in the home or landscape
- Understanding the influence of the past on the present
- Understanding the possibility of change

Activities

- Invite group members to cut out items that remind them of a place they used to live in.
- Include furniture, cupboards, interior and exterior objects.
- Use white glue to 'recreate' the environment on A4 paper.
- Share the picture.

Attachment Relevance

This exercise enables participants to connect with the past and create representations of that past.

This page may be photocopied for instructional use only. *Working with Attachment Difficulties in Teenagers* © Sue Jennings 2019

34 Houses 2

⦿ Individuals & groups

Resources

Old magazines and catalogues, scissors for each person, white glue and thick A4 paper.

Description

This exercise continues the idea of communicating about environments and relationships.

Learning Outcomes

- Expressing both people and places from the past
- Owning past experience
- Understanding the possibility for change
- Insight into personal life stories

Activities

- Suggest to participants that they recreate both an environment as well as the people there.
- Create a room or a building based on early experience.
- Cut out pictures of people that look like those that were in this space.
- Think about stories from this environment and share.

Attachment Relevance

Recreating echoes of people in a past environment helps to understand displaced or fractured relationships.

This page may be photocopied for instructional use only. *Working with Attachment Difficulties in Teenagers* © Sue Jennings 2019

35 Houses 3

⊙ Individuals & groups

Resources

Old magazines and catalogues, scissors for each person, white glue and thick A4 paper.

Description

This house exercise allows participants to think about change and the future, to plan the environment they would like to have.

Learning Outcomes

- Moving beyond the current situation
- Development of hope
- Acknowledgment of change
- Differentiating the future from the past

Activities

- Suggest the participants to move from the past to the future.
- Plan an environment they would like to live in.
- Choose the most important things that should be in the environment.
- Share with group members.

Attachment Relevance

This exercise encourages new beginnings, as well as enabling individual choice.

This page may be photocopied for instructional use only. *Working with Attachment Difficulties in Teenagers* © Sue Jennings 2019

36 House 4

⊙ Individuals & groups

Resources

Old magazines and catalogues, scissors for each person, white glue and thick A4 paper.

Description

Building on the ideas about houses in the previous activities, it is important to acknowledge that they are located in environments, near other houses.

Learning Outcomes

- Exploring the environment that people would choose to live in
- Allowing the proximity of other people
- Encouraging sociability
- Building self-esteem through possibilities

Activities

- Suggest participants think about the external world of their house.
- Where would it be located? How near are other houses?
- Who lives in them?
- Share individual perceptions of future 'worlds'.
- Share pictures.

Attachment Relevance

Encouraging a wider awareness of other people's worlds helps build greater security in the environment.

This page may be photocopied for instructional use only. *Working with Attachment Difficulties in Teenagers* © Sue Jennings 2019

37 Tissue Paper 1

⊙ Individuals & groups

Resources

Contrasting colours of tissue paper, white glue (diluted) and A4 paper.

Description

Through the use of torn paper, it is possible to move from a 'jagged' picture into something more rounded and fulfilling.

Learning Outcomes

- Putting pieces together
- Recognising that life can be fragmented, but can be mended
- Increasing awareness of art and healing
- Building confidence through fail-safe techniques

Activities

- Tear some pieces of tissue paper into rough circles a little larger than a pound coin.
- Choose contrasting colours.
- Stick them on A4 paper to create a picture.
- Use strips of tissue paper to create a frame around the picture.

Attachment Relevance

Framing the picture 'contains' the experience and sets boundaries.

This page may be photocopied for instructional use only. *Working with Attachment Difficulties in Teenagers* © Sue Jennings 2019

38 Tissue Paper 2

◉ Individuals & groups

Resources

Contrasting colours of tissue paper, white glue (diluted) and A4 paper; a paint brush for each person, coloured pens.

Description

Showing how torn and crumpled paper can be a mirror for experience.

Learning Outcomes

- Understanding that fractures can be mended
- Containment of experience
- Exploration of past into present
- Recognising that broken can mean beauty

Activities

- Tear up small pieces of tissue paper in contrasting colours.
- Paint diluted white glue all over the paper and sprinkle the pieces of tissue paper all over the A4 paper; allow it to dry.
- When dry, crumple the paper up and unfold it.
- Use a coloured pen to trace all the 'cracks'.

Attachment Relevance

This exercise develops a sense of being able to integrate previously fractured experiences.

This page may be photocopied for instructional use only. *Working with Attachment Difficulties in Teenagers* © Sue Jennings 2019

39 Tissue Paper 3

◉ Individuals & groups

Resources

Contrasting colours of tissue paper, white glue (diluted) and A4 paper; a paint brush for each person, coloured pens.

Description

Exploration of crumpled paper symbolising a 'messed up' life.

Learning Outcomes

- Owning previous experiences
- Trusting that the past can change in the future
- Confronting broken issues
- Discovering that broken images create art

Activities

- Encourage participants to choose two different colours of tissue paper.
- Crumple up a piece of tissue paper into a tight ball and let it unfold again.
- Smooth the paper out.
- Stick one piece on top of another.

Attachment Relevance

The smoothing of the past into a more tolerable future.

This page may be photocopied for instructional use only. *Working with Attachment Difficulties in Teenagers* © Sue Jennings 2019

40 Understanding My Brain 1

◉ Individuals & groups

Resources

Pieces of A4 paper and coloured pens; Worksheet 1, 'This is My Brain 1', for each person.

Description

Beginning to understand, in simple terms, the way the human brain works and the evolutionary processes that resulted in the reptilian brain, the mammalian (limbic) brain and the neocortex. (See the Introduction for an outline of brain areas, development and function.)

For this exercise we are thinking about the 'reptilian brain' and how it can sabotage what we do.

Learning Outcomes

- Understanding the instinctual brain
- Awareness of what is useful about this brain
- Awareness of what is not helpful about this part of the brain
- Developing an analytical mind to understand how the brain works

Activities

- Explain the working of the reptilian brain: that it reacts without primary thought.
- Identify the reptilian brain on the worksheet.
- Write down or draw aspects of myself that are governed by my instinctual/reptilian brain.
- Discuss whether these need to be changed.

Attachment Relevance

Understanding the several aspects of the brain, including the instinctual and the nurturing will help to repair attachments.

P This page may be photocopied for instructional use only. *Working with Attachment Difficulties in Teenagers* © Sue Jennings 2019

41 Understanding My Brain 2

⊙ Individuals & groups

Resources

Pieces of A4 paper and coloured pens; Worksheet 2, 'This is My Brain 2', for each person.

Description

Continuing the theme of how our brains work, this exercise helps us to understand the part of our brain we share with all other mammals, the mammalian (limbic) brain.

Learning Outcomes

- Understanding the nurturing aspect of our brains
- Awareness that it is shared by other mammals
- Developing an understanding that our ability to nurture is controlled by our brains
- Understanding the relationship between the reptilian brain and the mammalian brain

Activities

- Talk about the area of the brain that is shared by other mammals, and which is responsible for feelings and nurture.
- Colour in the mammalian brain on the worksheet.
- Draw or write down the aspects of your behaviour controlled by your mammalian brain.
- Share the relationship between the mammalian brain and the reptilian brain.

Attachment Relevance

It is important for teenagers to develop the capacity to nurture both themselves and others, which has often been neglected in the early attachment process.

This page may be photocopied for instructional use only. *Working with Attachment Difficulties in Teenagers* © Sue Jennings 2019

42 Understanding My Brain 3

⊙ Individuals & groups

Resources

Pieces of A4 paper and coloured pens; Worksheet 3, 'This is My Brain', for each person.

Description

Learning about the executive function (neocortex) of the brain enables teenagers to understand how they make decisions and choices.

Learning Outcomes

- Understanding the logical part of the brain
- Awareness of cognitive function
- Processing skills that belong to this part of the brain
- Contrasting it with other parts of the brain

Activities

- Explain how the executive function of the brain enables us to make decisions, reflect on choices and to pause before action.
- Colour that part of the brain on the worksheet.
- Draw or write down things that I make decisions about or need to think about.
- Consider how this part of the brain relates to the mammalian brain and the reptilian brain.

Attachment Relevance

Teenagers with attachment difficulties often have problems with decision-making and reflective thinking.

This page may be photocopied for instructional use only. *Working with Attachment Difficulties in Teenagers* © Sue Jennings 2019

43 Understanding My Brain 4

⊙ Groups
If working individually then the facilitator and child can have a puppet on each hand.

Resources

A set of glove puppets for each group of three, to represent the three areas of the brain: a snake for the reptilian brain, a cow for the mammalian brain and a boy and a girl for the executive function.

Description

Through the use of puppets, teenagers are able to understand contrasting aspects of their behaviour.

Learning Outcomes

- Awareness of contrasting brain function
- Communicating brain function through puppets
- Practical skills belonging to each brain aspect
- Deeper understanding of what controls behaviour

Activities

- In small groups of three, give each member a glove puppet representing one function of the brain.
- Remind them of the function of this puppet.
- Encourage the puppets to interact.
- Suggest a story could be created using these three puppets about instinctive behaviour, nurturing behaviour and reflective thinking.

Attachment Relevance

Teenagers are able to understand the way that these three aspects of their brains affect their behaviour, their feelings and their relationships.

This page may be photocopied for instructional use only. *Working with Attachment Difficulties in Teenagers* © Sue Jennings 2019

44 Understanding My Brain 5

⊙ Individuals & groups

Resources

Coloured pens; Worksheet 4, 'Inside My Head', for each person.

Description

It is important for teenagers to express what they feel is inside their brains.

Learning Outcomes

- Awareness of the dominant feelings that are inside my head
- Understanding how I communicate these feelings
- Developing skills at communicating in new ways
- Showing that behaviour can change

Activities

- Explain that people often keep things 'inside their heads' without expressing them.
- Colour in the worksheet using different colours for different feelings.
- Show which is the strongest feeling.
- Share with others how that feeling is usually expressed.

Attachment Relevance

Greater awareness of feelings and behaviour will contribute to longer lasting relationships.

This page may be photocopied for instructional use only. *Working with Attachment Difficulties in Teenagers* © Sue Jennings 2019

45 Understanding My Brain 6

◉ Individuals & groups

Resources

Coloured pens; Worksheet 5, 'Inside Your Head', for each person.

Description

Through understanding the thoughts and feelings of someone else, empathy can be created between individuals.

Learning Outcomes

- Awareness of empathy
- Communication of one's perceptions of other people
- Fine-tuning our understanding of others
- Readjusting our own projections

Activities

- Explain to the group that we are often misled about what others might be thinking or feeling.
- Using the worksheet, colour in what we feel somebody else is thinking and feeling.
- Discuss with a partner whether this is based on fact.
- Explain how easy it is to project onto other people, rather than to empathise with them.

Attachment Relevance

Teenagers learn to understand their own attachment behaviour by understanding their capacity to empathise.

This page may be photocopied for instructional use only. *Working with Attachment Difficulties in Teenagers* © Sue Jennings 2019

46 Who Do I Admire? 1

◉ Individuals & groups

Resources

Pens and coloured pencils; Worksheet 6, 'Who do I Admire?', for each person.

Description

Teenagers often copy role models of people whom they admire. It is important they develop an awareness of how they make these choices.

Learning Outcomes

- Developing awareness of people who set us an example
- Understanding how we choose the qualities we admire in other people
- Processing the relationship between helpful and unhelpful role models
- Understanding how people often behave like mirrors

Activities

- Discuss the worksheet with group members.
- Invite them to share qualities they admire in others and write them on the board.
- Colour the worksheet with emphasis on the most important qualities.
- General discussion about how we develop positive qualities.

Attachment Relevance

Often teenagers, when younger, were exposed to role models that are inappropriate; healthy attachments let us decide which qualities are positive for ourselves.

This page may be photocopied for instructional use only. *Working with Attachment Difficulties in Teenagers* © Sue Jennings 2019

47 Who Do I Admire? 2

⊙ Individuals & groups

Resources

A range of magazines, scissors for each person, white glue, thick paper and coloured pens.

Description

Many people we admire are famous people, past and present. By identifying their qualities we develop a greater understanding of ourselves.

Learning Outcomes

- Understanding clearly the way that we are attracted to other people
- Developing a sixth sense about our own intuition
- Owning when some qualities are not right for ourselves
- Acknowledging our personal capacity for change and maturing

Activities

- Explain to the group that they can create a collage of people whom they admire.
- Cut out pictures from magazines representing these people – either individuals, or possibly those who represent a 'type'.
- Stick them on a collage and colour in any spaces.
- Share with a partner.

Attachment Relevance

The capacity to integrate positive qualities from other people helps us to build self-esteem.

This page may be photocopied for instructional use only. *Working with Attachment Difficulties in Teenagers* © Sue Jennings 2019

48 My Favourite YouTube 1

⊙ Individuals & groups

Resources

Access to a working computer and internet connection.

Description

It is important to respond to a teenager's enjoyment of YouTube videos, and allow them to make choices.

Learning Outcomes

- Creating a relationship through a shared video
- Identifying personal likes and dislikes
- Developing language skills of description
- Developing confidence to express personal preferences

Activities

- Discuss with the individual or group favourite YouTube videos.
- Encourage words that describe how we feel about these videos.
- Share one with the group.
- Discuss it afterwards.

Attachment Relevance

Allowing choices and decision-making help to develop an attachment relationship.

P This page may be photocopied for instructional use only. *Working with Attachment Difficulties in Teenagers* © Sue Jennings 2019

49 My Favourite YouTube 2

⊙ Individuals & groups

Resources

Access to a working computer and internet connection; each person to have a smartphone, if possible.

Description

This activity is similar to Activity 48, but the aim is to identify even more things that are liked or disliked about YouTube videos.

Learning Outcomes

- Development of the language of choice
- Being able to express likes and dislikes
- Understanding contrast of preferences (rather than a generalised response)
- Encouraging personal opinions that may be different from those of others

Activities

- Continue the discussion about the variety of YouTube videos.
- Pose the question, 'If I made something for YouTube, what would it be about?'
- Invite each group member to film 30 seconds of something important to them, using a smart phone.
- Share the clips.

Attachment Relevance

Building confidence through making choices and being able to create something as an individual.

This page may be photocopied for instructional use only. *Working with Attachment Difficulties in Teenagers* © Sue Jennings 2019

50 My Favourite YouTube 3

⊙ Groups

Resources

Access to a working computer and internet connection; each person to have a smartphone, if possible.

Description

Encourage creativity through making a brief video.

Learning Outcomes

- Appreciating the art form of video-making
- Understanding that visual images can be fine-tuned, just the same as paintings or clay models
- Developing appreciation of the art of self and others
- The capacity to accept constructive criticism

Activities

- Encourage the group to work in pairs and design a video episode, a maximum of 2 minutes long.
- Suggest they can film on location away from the activity centre.
- Allow enough time for them to come back and share images.
- Discuss similarities and differences

Attachment Relevance

Continuing to build self-esteem through the development of successful artwork.

This page may be photocopied for instructional use only. *Working with Attachment Difficulties in Teenagers* © Sue Jennings 2019

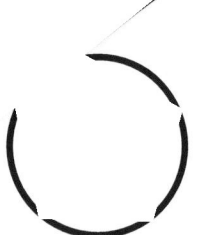

My Favourite YouTube 4

⊙ Groups

Resources

A rolling 'internet programme' created with the short video clips of group members; pieces of card and coloured pens.

Description

After the development of individual and small group filming, this exercise puts several pieces together to create a mini festival.

Learning Outcomes

- Application of critical standards to creativity
- Understanding a range of choices in the art forms of the festival
- Valuing personal contribution to a personal project
- The ability to constructively criticise different exhibits

Activities

- View and discuss the various contributions for the mini festival.
- Create titles for the various videos.
- Make a programme for the videos in the festival, using the card and coloured pens.
- Share all the exhibits and note any commentary on the programme.

Where appropriate, invite other people to see the video clips of participants.

Attachment Relevance

This exercise is a culmination of confidence building and creativity that is being share, not only with one other person, but also with members of the community.

This page may be photocopied for instructional use only. *Working with Attachment Difficulties in Teenagers* © Sue Jennings 2019

52 Games Console 1

⦿ Individual & groups

Resources

Games console and controller; the group leader must have experience in playing Minecraft or Terraria.

Description

Using internet gaming, teenagers can communicate past and future experience.

Learning Outcomes

- The familiarity of the internet encourages confidence
- Developing greater communication skills
- Moving on from negative experience
- Differentiating life experiences

Activities

- Discuss how these video games can be used to communicate personal experience.
- Using Minecraft, invite group members to recreate an unhappy time in their past.
- Build the environment and the people involved.
- Share with the group or a partner.

Attachment Relevance

Encourage teenagers to communicate their past experiences and to share safely with others.

This page may be photocopied for instructional use only. *Working with Attachment Difficulties in Teenagers* © Sue Jennings 2019

53 Games Console 2

⊙ Individual & groups

Resources

Games console and controller; the group leader must have experience in playing Minecraft or Terraria.

Description

In contrast with Activity 52, this exercise builds on positive experiences.

Learning Outcomes

- Developing a feeling of control over one's own destiny
- Understanding that our chosen life paths may have different outcomes
- Supporting other group members in their ideas and planning
- Refining our own ideas of what we do with our lives

Activities

- Discuss with the group how they can create present or future experiences.
- Suggest group members remember positive experiences and then go on to build on these.
- Use Minecraft to create a whole new world in terms of environment and people.
- Make sure that group members do not use the violent images.

Attachment Relevance

Using the Minecraft game to create positive possibilities and a decrease in negative influences.

This page may be photocopied for instructional use only. *Working with Attachment Difficulties in Teenagers* © Sue Jennings 2019

54 Games Console 3

◉ Individual & groups

Resources

Games console and controller; the group leader must have experience in playing Minecraft or Terraria.

Description

Further use of Minecraft can enable teenagers to be more creative in fashioning their own world.

Learning Outcomes

- Introducing the idea of hope for people who have had troubled lives
- Allowing group members to experiment with creating worlds
- Encouraging teenagers to have a stress-free environment
- Supporting group members in individual choice, at the same time as group sharing

Activities

- Encourage the addition of greater detail while creating a new world with Minecraft.
- Remind participants that they are creating a world without stress.
- Allow time for experimentation before finishing their world.
- Share ideas and images.

Attachment Relevance

Group members are making positive decisions about their futures.

This page may be photocopied for instructional use only. *Working with Attachment Difficulties in Teenagers* © Sue Jennings 2019

55 Important Images 1

⊙ Individual & groups

Resources

A variety of colour magazines, scissors for each person, white glue and card.

Description

Participants look at magazines, select photographs that they find pleasing, and use these photographs to create a montage.

Learning Outcomes

- Personal decisions regarding visual images
- Understanding that there are different ways to perceive our world
- Creating a blend of different images
- Getting in touch with personal significance

Activities

- Give people time to look at the magazines, choose pictures and cut them up.
- Arrange the pictures on card to create a montage.
- Draw a frame around the montage.
- Share the picture with others.

Attachment Relevance

Putting together contrasting images helps to transform fragmented relationships.

P This page may be photocopied for instructional use only. *Working with Attachment Difficulties in Teenagers* © Sue Jennings 2019

56 Important Images 2

⊙ Individual & groups

Resources

Access to outdoors, if possible; camera or smartphone for each person; a printer and paper; card for making frames.

Description

Participants are encouraged to choose indoor or outdoor images to photograph, then to create frames and share their images.

Learning Outcomes

- Making choices between visual images
- Building confidence through camera or smartphone use
- Contrasting shapes and colours
- Non-verbal communication with others.

Activities

- Explain to the group that they have a choice of images to record.
- Give time outside and inside for people to take up to six pictures.
- Review the pictures and choose one to share; print it out and create a frame around it.
- Share the images.

Attachment Relevance

Building confidence through communicating images to others.

This page may be photocopied for instructional use only. *Working with Attachment Difficulties in Teenagers* © Sue Jennings 2019

57 Important Images 3

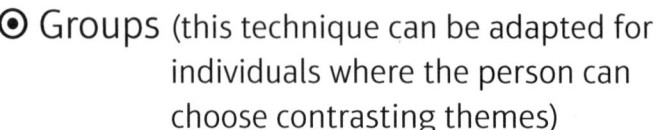

⦿ Groups (this technique can be adapted for individuals where the person can choose contrasting themes)

Resources

Access to outdoors; camera or smartphone for each person; a printer and paper; display board for an exhibition.

Description

Several people work together and choose photographs to make their own exhibition.

Learning Outcomes

- Cooperation with others
- Decision-making
- Allowing others to contribute
- Taking pleasure in the whole, rather than the individual parts

Activities

- Group members work in pairs and take contrasting pictures of different outdoor images.
- Decide which images are suitable for the exhibition.
- Plan with other group members the arrangement of the photographs.
- Create the group exhibition.

Attachment Relevance

Participants are learning to work together and trust other people in decision-making.

This page may be photocopied for instructional use only. *Working with Attachment Difficulties in Teenagers* © Sue Jennings 2019

58 Important Images 4

◉ Groups
This techniques can be adapted around contrasting themes for individuals.

Resources

Camera or smartphone for each person; a printer and paper; display board for an exhibition.

Description

This exercise encourages taking portraits of each other (or selfies), working with another individual and creating a portrait gallery to display.

Learning Outcomes

- Building confidence by creating a portrait
- Risk-taking by displaying a self-portrait
- Understanding how to observe and comment
- Accepting observations from others

Activities

- Explain to group members they are going to create a portrait gallery.
- Work in pairs to take photographs of each other.
- Experiment with a straight portrait and a 'quirky' portrait.
- Display the pictures as a portrait gallery.

Photography can also be used in later role-plays when groups are playing in costume.

Attachment Relevance

This exercise builds trust between two people to create portraits that can be displayed.

P This page may be photocopied for instructional use only. *Working with Attachment Difficulties in Teenagers* © Sue Jennings 2019

59 Group Painting

⊙ Groups

Resources

Large piece of card or thick paper for the whole group to work on; paints, paintbrushes and coloured pens.

Description

This exercise makes connections between internet images and the sensory world of art.

Learning Outcomes

- Group collaboration
- Tolerance of other people's ideas
- Understanding one's own symbolic space on the paper
- Communication between group members

Activities

- Invite people to remember the different images they created through Minecraft in Activities 53 and 54.
- Create a group picture of their favourite Minecraft images.
- Make sure everyone's ideas are included.
- Share and talk about the images.

Attachment Relevance

Building relationships through group painting.

This page may be photocopied for instructional use only. *Working with Attachment Difficulties in Teenagers* © Sue Jennings 2019

60 Individual Painting

⊙ Individuals

Resources

Large piece of card or thick paper; paints, paintbrush and coloured pens.

Description

Encouraging individuals to develop their Minecraft experiences into a montage.

Learning Outcomes

- Integrating internet images into a reality montage
- Exercising personal choices of colour and shape
- Experiencing personal positive attitude and removing negative attitude
- Encouragement of communication through art

Activities

- Encourage the individual to describe their positive images from Minecraft developed in Activities 53 and 54.
- Create a montage through painting and drawing these previous images.
- Think of a title that accurately sums up feelings of this picture.
- Share and discuss.

Attachment Relevance

Continuing to develop positive attachment through creativity.

This page may be photocopied for instructional use only. *Working with Attachment Difficulties in Teenagers* © Sue Jennings 2019

Part 3
Drama: Roles, Scenes & Solutions

For some teenagers with attachment difficulties the activities in this section can be challenging without sufficient grounding. The previous two sections allow for the development of self-confidence and self-worth and encourage affirmation through creativity. Without this affirmation, role-techniques are often avoided, as they can feel unsafe. On the other hand, some participants do gain from being able to play the role of someone they wish to emulate.

Generally speaking, however, young people will build the confidence for role-playing by being able to embody the qualities of a role or character. This will be enhanced by the embodiment techniques in Part 1 (particularly Activities 18 to 30), and then consolidated by the projective techniques in Part 2.

Warm-up games increase physical confidence and expression of feelings in a structured form; again we are creating forms that 'contain without restraint'. The aim is to facilitate the expression of feelings without these becoming overwhelming.

With grounding in the games, participants will feel more confident to create scenes that can then be improvised and enacted. Newspaper headlines are invaluable here, as they provide ready-made situations that can be explored through role-play – with or without words. Props, such as a piece of cloth, can be used to stimulate ideas for improvisation.

After the warm-ups and improvisations there follow several scenes taken from Shakespeare's plays, which address family relationships in a safe structure. There are very powerful emotions in these dialogues that can be enacted, discussed, and then explored in different ways. For example, is an angry father more frightening when he shouts or when he expresses the words in quiet anger, even in an angry whisper?

This section closes with some dragon exploration, which leads into the integrated themes in Part 4.

Warm-Up Games 1

) Individuals & groups

Resources

Suitable space for drama.

Description

In this activity participants express thoughts and feelings physically, as well as managing themselves in space.

Learning Outcomes

- Experiencing a range of emotions
- Physical coordination in space
- Consolidation of drama skills for role-play
- Insight into how other people feel

Activities

- Invite participants to walk briskly round the room, then run, then walk very slowly.
- Explain that whenever 'freeze' is called the participants stand absolutely still.
- Explain that whenever 'freeze' is called everyone has to stop and express a shape with their body: round, tall, thin, spiky, twisted.
- Continue this exercise with variations of shape to develop greater flexibility.

Attachment Relevance

Building up the body-self, in order to feel physically confident.

This page may be photocopied for instructional use only. *Working with Attachment Difficulties in Teenagers* © Sue Jennings 2019

62 Warm-Up Games 2

⊙ Individuals & groups

Resources

Suitable space for drama.

Description

Developing confidence in space, with movement and sound as a preparation for drama.

Learning Outcomes

- Fine-tuning physical responses
- Spatial awareness and self-control
- Understanding the amount of space that people feel necessary between themselves and others.
- Developing interpersonal reactions

Activities

- Explain that participants can be more adventurous in their movement and develop greater spatial awareness.
- Walk briskly around the room and freeze in a role: old person, child, teacher and policeman.
- Add facial expression and hand gestures to the roles.
- Create a body-sculpt in pairs, with each person in a different role, for example: teenager and policeman, or woman and child. Individuals may work with the facilitator

Attachment Relevance

Developing emotional expression through everyday roles and relationships.

This page may be photocopied for instructional use only. *Working with Attachment Difficulties in Teenagers* © Sue Jennings 2019

63 Warm-Up Games 3

⊙ Individuals & groups

Resources

Suitable space for drama.

Description

Participants prepare for more complex understanding of roles.

Learning Outcomes

- Developing empathy and understanding
- Understanding the importance of sharing feelings
- Improving emotional intelligence
- Encouraging non-verbal communication

Activities

- Walk briskly around the room and 'freeze' into shapes at the call of 'freeze'.
- Allow the shapes transform into roles; each person follows their own inclination as to role.
- Assign feelings to the roles, such as angry child, patient teacher, irritated policeman or woman.
- Encourage various characters to interact in pairs – individuals may interact with the facilitator.

Attachment Relevance

It is important to encourage the development of empathy as part of the attachment process.

This page may be photocopied for instructional use only. *Working with Attachment Difficulties in Teenagers* © Sue Jennings 2019

64 Warm-Up Games 4

⊙ Groups

Resources

Suitable space for drama; pieces of paper with different emotions written on them, such as angry, sad, irritable, scared, and so on; a second set of pieces of paper with roles, such as teacher, mother, grandma, child and train driver, and so on.

Description

Developing brief scenes out of the roles.

Learning Outcomes

- Development of roles in detail
- Appropriate interaction with others
- Understanding how others feel
- Containment of role boundaries

Activities

- Focus energy by everyone running around the room, weaving in and out between other people.
- Invite participants to choose a role and an emotion and think about how they will put them together.
- Give time for them to practise walking with physical and facial expressions.
- People work in pairs, in their roles, interacting in a small scene.

Attachment Relevance

Developing role flexibility and emotional intelligence.

This page may be photocopied for instructional use only. *Working with Attachment Difficulties in Teenagers* © Sue Jennings 2019

65 Warm-Up Games 5

⊙ Groups

Resources

Suitable space for drama; pieces of paper with the roles and emotions first used in Activity 64.

Description

Developing further brief scenes out of the roles first encountered in Activity 64.

Learning Outcomes

- Development of roles in detail
- Appropriate interaction with others
- Understanding how others feel
- Containment of role boundaries

Activities

- Warm-up with everyone walking around the room.
- Invite people to form into twos or threes.
- Everyone chooses a roles and emotion.
- Develop a scene in which the three characters interact with each other.

Attachment Relevance

Increased confidence in role flexibility contributes to healthy attachments and relationships.

This page may be photocopied for instructional use only. *Working with Attachment Difficulties in Teenagers* © Sue Jennings 2019

66 Newspaper Themes 1

⊙ Groups
This technique can be adapted for individuals.

Resources

Suitable space for drama; a number of short news headlines from a range of newspapers and magazines, or social media. These need to involve two or three people and an adult or adult/child relationship. For example: 'Man jailed for domestic violence', or 'Missing child found safe'.

Description

This exercise works with real stories from the media and encourages exploration of different perspectives.

Learning Outcomes

- Increased empathy
- Social and cultural awareness
- Understanding different perspectives
- Different outcomes and solutions

Activities

- Invite pairs to choose one headline and discuss what the story might involve.
- Create a role-play that is relevant to the headline.
- Experiment with endings relevant to the headline.
- Choose one to show other group members.

Attachment Relevance

Dramatic improvisations about relationships help to strengthen positive attachments.

This page may be photocopied for instructional use only. *Working with Attachment Difficulties in Teenagers* © Sue Jennings 2019

67 Newspaper Themes 2

◉ Individuals

Resources

Cut out a selection of 'feeling' words from newspapers and magazines, such as happy, bored, angry, surprised, scared, startled, content, and so on; A4 paper, white glue.

Description

This exercise supports a teenager who struggles to communicate their feelings.

Learning Outcomes

- Identifying feelings
- Expressing feelings
- Linking feelings to actions
- Relevant mood change

Activities

- Encourage the teenager to think about their different feelings.
- Choose words that represent their most frequent feelings.
- Stick the words with white glue onto the paper.
- Share the different feelings and when they are felt.

Attachment Relevance

Teenagers who are securely attached are able to express a range of emotions in response to given situations.

This page may be photocopied for instructional use only. *Working with Attachment Difficulties in Teenagers* © Sue Jennings 2019

68 Newspaper Themes 3

⊙ Individuals & groups

Resources

A4 white card, one sheet per person, divided into 4 equal spaces; a number of cut-out newspaper or magazine headlines, coloured pens.

Description

This exercise encourages reflection on social situations and allowing for individual differences.

Learning Outcomes

- Greater social awareness
- Increased understanding of others' viewpoints
- Problem solving
- Choice of solutions

Activities

- Explain to group members that in the first square they will stick a headline of their own choice.
- They ask themselves what happened next, and write or draw it in square number 2.
- In square number 3, write or draw anyone else who was involved.
- In square number 4, write or draw how it ended.

Attachment Relevance

Teenagers are developing a greater self and social awareness, which is important in healthy attachments.

This page may be photocopied for instructional use only. *Working with Attachment Difficulties in Teenagers* © Sue Jennings 2019

69 Newspaper Themes 4

⊙ Individuals and groups

Resources

Choice of short newspaper stories with headlines.

Description

Participants are encouraged to discuss and encourage possible solutions to a conflict story.

Learning Outcomes

- Understanding similarities and differences
- Listening to other perspectives
- Understanding choices
- Making informed decisions

Activities

- Invite group members to form small groups. Individuals can work with the facilitator.
- Each group chooses a story to explore.
- Discuss the important issues in the story.
- Use drama to explore potential outcomes.

Attachment Relevance

Teenagers are developing a greater self and social awareness, which is important in healthy attachments.

This page may be photocopied for instructional use only. *Working with Attachment Difficulties in Teenagers* © Sue Jennings 2019

70 Newspaper Themes 5

⦿ Individuals & groups

Resources

Pens, coloured pencils, A4 card or thick paper.

Description

Participants imagine they are in the role of a journalist and create a story they would like to explore.

Learning Outcomes

- Developing curiosity
- Discovering facts
- Encouraging communication skills
- Making choices

Activities

- Ask the group to form pairs and explore a story by means of an interview: one person plays the journalist and the other the person being interviewed. Individuals may work with the facilitator.
- Decide what the story is about.
- Assist the 'journalist' with a series of prompts that can be written on the board, for example: Where, When, How and Who.
- Role-play the interview and write a brief newspaper article.

Attachment Relevance

Increased awareness of others helps to develop empathy.

This page may be photocopied for instructional use only. *Working with Attachment Difficulties in Teenagers* © Sue Jennings 2019

71 Improvisation through Objects

⦿ Individuals & groups

Resources

A collection of objects in a box or basket to stimulate ideas, for example: postcards from holiday destinations, an old wallet with old cards and money, an hourglass with sand, an old-fashioned small clock, a picture of a ship, and so on. The objects should be very varied and mainly within the life experience of the teenagers.

Description

Improvisation around a chosen object enables storytelling and then dramatisation.

Learning Outcomes

- Stimulating association and ideas
- Creative thinking
- Thinking about objects and their relationships
- Making life drama connections

Activities

- Explain the exercise to individuals or the group.
- Invite them to choose an object and think about it.
- Create a short story about the object and its significance.
- Dramatise the story with other group members. (Optional, the story telling may be sufficient.)

Attachment Relevance

Stimulation of the imagination and personal memories can further strengthen relationships.

This page may be photocopied for instructional use only. *Working with Attachment Difficulties in Teenagers* © Sue Jennings 2019

72 Improvisation through Pictures 1

⊙ Individuals & groups

Resources

A collection of picture postcards, showing a variety of buildings.

Description

Using postcards depicting buildings, individuals or small groups are encouraged to make associations and imagine a scenario relating to the building. Paper, pens, coloured pencils.

Learning Outcomes

- Improving skills in choice and decision-making
- Stimulation of creativity
- Recognition of past environments
- Free association of ideas

Activities

- Invite the teenagers to examine the postcards and choose one.
- Reflect on possible ideas about the place.
- Think of an incident that happened in or outside one of the buildings.
- Write or draw a short story about this scene.

Attachment Relevance

It is important for teenagers to create attachment understanding with places as well as people.

This page may be photocopied for instructional use only. *Working with Attachment Difficulties in Teenagers* © Sue Jennings 2019

73 Improvisation through Pictures 2

⊙ Individuals & groups

Resources

Story material from Activity 72, or further use of postcards; hand puppets.

Description

The story from the previous activity can be used for role-play and creating dramatic scenes.

Learning Outcomes

- Understanding how stories are dramatised
- Expansion of ideas
- Sharing ideas with others
- Improvisation into dramatic structure

Activities

- Small groups or individuals work with hand puppets.
- Discuss everyone's stories about the different buildings.
- Choose a story as a theme for the drama (or a combination of themes).
- Create a drama from the story and perform it with hand puppets for other group members.

Attachment Relevance

Continuing relevant attachment to places and past events.

This page may be photocopied for instructional use only. *Working with Attachment Difficulties in Teenagers* © Sue Jennings 2019

74 Improvisation through Costume

⊙ Individuals and Groups

Resources

A collection of hats and scarfs, including flat cap, top hat, bonnet, beanie hat, balaclava, fancy hat with flowers, trilby, fedora, and so on.

Description

Developing role-plays using simple costumes helps to develop a deeper understanding of characters and their feelings. If working with an individual, the facilitator can participate 'in role' themselves.

Learning Outcomes

- Deeper understanding of characters and roles.
- Awareness of others in a situation.
- Sharing of ideas (generosity).
- Developing critical awareness.

Activities

- Experiment with choosing a hat and walking across the room in character.
- Explore several hats and walks before choosing one.
- Greet other people in the group as the character of your hat.
- Create drama improvisations in small groups.

Attachment Relevance

In-depth exploration of individuals and their characteristics is important in resolving attachment issues.

This page may be photocopied for instructional use only. *Working with Attachment Difficulties in Teenagers* © Sue Jennings 2019

75 Improvisation using Fabric

⊙ Individuals and Groups

Resources

Different textures and sizes of fabric, for example: green baize (pool tables), length of white net, pieces of see-through chiffon, fur fabric, shawls and ponchos.

Description

Using lengths of cloth to either create environments or simple costumes.

Learning Outcomes

- Wider expansion of themes with greater detail
- Collaboration with others in creation
- Shared responsibility of outcomes
- Decision-making over structure and outcome

Activities

- Encourage group members to create environments using the fabric over chairs and tables.
- In small groups, choose an environment for a mystery play;
- Choose the characters and improvise, leading into a dramatised scene.
- Share with others

Attachment Relevance

In-depth exploration of individuals and their characteristics is important in resolving attachment issues.

This page may be photocopied for instructional use only. *Working with Attachment Difficulties in Teenagers* © Sue Jennings 2019

76 Role Play: Girlfriends

⊙ Groups

Resources

Any props required for the characters; Worksheet 7, 'Shakespeare Role-Play: Girlfriends', for each person.

Description

A brief scene from Shakespeare's *A Midsummer Night's Dream* (Act I, scene 1) illustrates the reality of teenage friendships. In this extract Hermia and Helena are arguing over the same potential boyfriend.

Learning Outcomes

- Addresses actual teenage conflicts
- Encourages learning through 'distanced' experience
- Develops use of metaphor
- Allows conflict resolution

Activities

- Share the story of *A Midsummer Night's Dream*, or perhaps watch a DVD.
- Warm-up with game of 'catch', or a throw ball to other members of the group, calling out their name as you throw.
- In pairs, everyone reads through the dialogue.
- Experiment with movement, gestures, tone of voice; then change roles.

Hermia: I frown upon him, yet he loves me still.

Helena: Oh, that your frowns would teach my smiles such skill!

Hermia: I give him curses, yet he gives me love.

Helena: Oh, that my prayers could such affection move!

Hermia: The more I hate, the more he follows me.

Helena: The more I love, the more he hateth me.

Hermia: His folly, Helena, is no fault of mine.

Helena: None, but your beauty. Would that fault were mine!

Attachment Relevance

Teenage attachments are very important during maturation and the role-play addresses issues in a safe way.

This page may be photocopied for instructional use only. *Working with Attachment Difficulties in Teenagers* © Sue Jennings 2019

77 Role Play: Father & Daughter

◉ Individuals and Groups

Resources

Worksheet 8, 'Shakespeare Role Play: Father & Daughter', for each person; possible props for characters.

Description

A scene from *Romeo and Juliet* (Act III, scene v) between Juliet and her father and mother illustrates the dilemma of controlling parents. If working with an individual, the facilitator can participate 'in role'.

Learning Outcomes

- Stimulates discussion on teenage marriage
- Illustrates violent parental relationships
- Maintains a safe distance through using text
- Insight into family dynamics

Activities

- Share the story of *Romeo and Juliet*, or perhaps watch a DVD.
- Warm-up game of simulated tennis in pairs.
- Using the worksheets, read the dialogue in pairs. Juliet's mother is present and following the exchange between her husband and daughter, therefore the group could work in threes, if they wish, and swap roles.
- Explore movement, gestures, silent communication; change roles.

Juliet [to her mother]: I wonder at this haste, that I must wed
Ere he, that should be husband, comes to woo.
I pray you tell my lord and father, madam,
I will not marry yet …

Father: … Mistress minion you,
Thank me no thankings, nor proud me no prouds,
But fettle your fine joints 'gainst Thursday next
To go with Paris to Saint Peter's Church,
Or I will drag thee on a hurdle thither …

Attachment Relevance

Teenagers get 'stuck' in the communication with parents and confrontation is not always the best solution!

This page may be photocopied for instructional use only. *Working with Attachment Difficulties in Teenagers* © Sue Jennings 2019

78 Role Play: King & Helper

⊙ Groups

Resources

Worksheet 9, 'Shakespeare Role-Play: King & Helper', for each person; simple props or costumes.

Description

A scene from *A Midsummer Night's Dream* (Act III, scene ii) between Oberon and Puck, in which Puck has made an enormous mistake.

Learning Outcomes

- Encourages discussion of authority
- Illustrates magical world
- Maintains safe distance through using text
- Insight into authority and relationships

Activities

- Share the story of *A Midsummer Night's Dream*, or perhaps watch a DVD.
- Warm-up game keeping balloons in the air.
- Read the dialogue on the worksheet in pairs.
- Experiment with voice, gesture and movement.

Oberon: What hast thou done? Thou hast mistaken quite,
And laid the love juice on some true love's sight.
Of thy misprision must perforce ensue
Some true love turned, and not a false turned true.

Puck: Then fate o'errules that, one man holding troth
A million fail, confounding oath on oath.

Oberon: About the wood go swifter than the wind,
And Helena of Athens look thou find –
… By some illusion see thou bring her here.
I'll charm his eyes against she do appear.

Puck: I go, I go. Look how I go,
Swifter than arrow from the Tartar's bow.

Attachment Relevance

Exploration of relationships strengthens attachments.

This page may be photocopied for instructional use only. *Working with Attachment Difficulties in Teenagers* © Sue Jennings 2019

79 Role-Play: Chorus (*Henry V*)

⊙ Individuals & groups

Resources

Worksheet 10, 'Shakespeare Role-Play: Chorus (*Henry V*)' for each person; possible props for characters.

Description

A short speech by the Chorus who open *Henry V* (Act I, Prologue) to improve confidence and voice; this activity can be used with an individual or a small group taking a line each.

Learning Outcomes

- Encourages confidence through vocal exercises
- Illustrates the importance of imagery and metaphor
- Maintains safe distance through using text
- Encourages creating and exploring

Activities

- Share the story of *Henry V*, or perhaps watch a DVD.
- Warm-up game of simulated jousting in pairs.
- Read the dialogue on the worksheet in different ways: quickly, slowly, loudly, softly.
- Explore movement, gestures, silent communication.

Chorus: O for a muse of fire, that would ascend
The brightest heaven of invention,
A kingdom for a stage, princes to act
And monarchs to behold the swelling scene!
Then should the warlike Harry, like himself,
Assume the port of Mars; and at his heels,
Leash'd in like hounds, should famine, sword and fire
Crouch for employment.

Attachment Relevance

Teenagers need to build confidence and authority, and really enjoy creative activities.

This page may be photocopied for instructional use only. *Working with Attachment Difficulties in Teenagers* © Sue Jennings 2019

80 Role-Play: Lovers

⊙ Groups

Resources

Worksheet 11, 'Shakespeare Role-Play: Lovers', for each person; possible props for characters.

Description

Two separate extracts from the first act of *Twelfth Night* by Orsino and Viola illustrate the power of imagery in speaking of love.

Learning Outcomes

- Understanding the poetry of love
- Illustrates overwhelming feelings
- Maintains a safe distance through using text
- Insight into creativity through verse

Activities

- Share story of Twelfth Night, or perhaps watch a DVD.
- Warm-up game of deep breathing and running.
- Using the worksheet and working in pairs, each person takes one role and delivers their speech to the other. Remind the group that this is not a dialogue between these two people.
- Explore movement, gestures, changes in tone of voice; swap roles.

Orsino: If music be the food of love, play on;
Give me excess of it that, surfeiting,
The appetite may sicken and so die.
That strain again, it had a dying fall;
O it came o'er my ear like the sweet sound
That breathes upon a bank of violets,
Stealing and giving odour.

Act I, scene i

Viola: Make me a willow cabin at your gate,
And call upon my soul within the house,
Write loyal cantons of contemnèd love
And sing them loud even in the dead of night;

Act I, scene v

Attachment Relevance

Expressing feelings of love in an emergent relationship.

This page may be photocopied for instructional use only. *Working with Attachment Difficulties in Teenagers* © Sue Jennings 2019

81 Locks & Keys 1

⊙ Individuals & groups

Resources

A collection of different keys: large and small, door keys, treasure-box keys, and so on. Thick paper and pens.

Description

The symbol of the key suggests that a door may be opened or prevented from opening. It is an important metaphor for understanding a teenager's needs.

Learning Outcomes

- Exploring opening and closure
- Grasping that some doors may never be opened
- Following the beginning of a new idea
- Empowering the individual to ''own' the key

Activities

- Encourage everybody to explore all the keys and then to choose one.
- Draw around the key on the paper.
- Think what this key will open.
- Draw a picture of where this key will fit and describe what is inside.

Attachment Relevance

Finding metaphors to encourage teenagers to form attachments.

This page may be photocopied for instructional use only. *Working with Attachment Difficulties in Teenagers* © Sue Jennings 2019

82 Locks & Keys 2

◉ Individuals & groups

Resources

A collection of different keys, large and small, door keys, treasure-box keys, and so on; actual locks or pictures of locks. Thick paper and pens.

Description

The feeling of being locked out is an important metaphor for teenagers, whether they are excluded from a class, or their family, or their peer group.

Learning Outcomes

- Understanding exclusion
- Encouraging appropriate means to overcome the exclusion
- Associating feelings about inclusion and exclusion
- Understanding that inclusion could be frightening

Activities

- Encourage the participants to consider the different locks and those they might like to own. Draw one that is significant.
- Think of a situation where they feel locked out.
- Share with a partner and create physically not being allowed to enter.
- Create the opposite situation, in which someone is welcomed and allowed in.

Attachment Relevance

'Good enough' attachment includes feelings of inclusion.

83 Locks & Keys 3

⊙ Individuals & groups

Resources

Pictures of fairy-tale castles and palaces; drawing materials and paper.

Description

Building a fairy story around the idea of the castle.

Learning Outcomes

- Developing story-making skills
- Understanding the metaphors in stories
- Developing creative skills
- Enabling the development of a flexible voice

Activities

- Using the resource pictures, everyone develops their own image of a castle.
- Draw and colour the castle, but create a locked door, or drawbridge, or moat.
- Tell the story of this locked castle and who or what is being kept in or out.
- Suggest whether or not there is a rescuer.

Attachment Relevance

The metaphor of the locked door or building is often a metaphor for a teenager's personal experience.

This page may be photocopied for instructional use only. *Working with Attachment Difficulties in Teenagers* © Sue Jennings 2019

84 Locks & Keys 4

◉ Individuals & groups

Resources

Crayons, coloured pencils/pens and paper; Story Sheet 1, 'The Story of Rapunzel' & Worksheet 12, 'Rapunzel 1', one of each for everyone. You may expand this activity using Worksheets 13 & 14, 'Rapunzel 2' & 'Rapunzel 3', if it seems appropriate.

Description

Using the story of Rapunzel is a very useful metaphor for teenagers to be able to understand and escape from abuse.

Learning Outcomes

- Personal development through metaphor
- Finding resolution through a story
- Personal connections with old stories
- Empowering the self to change inevitability

Activities

- Each person has a copy of the story sheet.
- Read the story out loud and discuss.
- Using Worksheet 12, everyone creates their own picture of the tower in which Rapunzel was imprisoned.
- Consider the costumes that Rapunzel, the witch and the prince might wear.

If it seems appropriate, expand the activity by giving everyone copies of Worksheets 13 and 14 to fill in and colour.

Attachment Relevance

This continues the theme of being locked away and its relevance for teenage attachment.

This page may be photocopied for instructional use only. *Working with Attachment Difficulties in Teenagers* © Sue Jennings 2019

85 Locks & Keys 5

⊙ Individuals & groups

Resources

Coloured pens/pencils and paper.

Description

Encouraging teenagers to talk about experiences that should be locked away and those that need to be explored.

Learning Outcomes

- Learning the difference between what needs to be locked away and what needs to be explored
- Introducing the theme of forgiveness
- Making connections between what pulls us down and what moves us forward
- Developing autonomy over our own experiences

Activities

- Encourage discussion with the group about what needs to be forgiven and what needs to be locked away.
- Invite group members to draw a locked box and an open box.
- Colour in the boxes and describe their contents using metaphor.
- Think of a gift to give other members of the group, which can be put in their open treasure box.

Attachment Relevance

It is important for developing healthy attachment to be able to let go of negative experience.

This page may be photocopied for instructional use only. *Working with Attachment Difficulties in Teenagers* © Sue Jennings 2019

86 Dragons 1

◉ Individuals & groups

Resources

Pictures or postcards of different sorts of dragons; coloured pens/pencils and paper.

Description

Introducing the theme of the dragon enables teenagers to safely express a range of emotions, including anger.

Learning Outcomes

- Using metaphor to express angry feelings
- Creating stories that allow emotions to be expressed
- Greater insight into personal feelings
- Developing understanding of other people's angry feelings

Activities

- Discuss and explore the theme of dragons.
- Share any dragon stories group members may know.
- Draw one's own personal dragon.
- Colour it and draw a frame around it.

Attachment Relevance

Dragons represent a larger-than-life monster that teenagers can recognise and overcome to experience success.

This page may be photocopied for instructional use only. *Working with Attachment Difficulties in Teenagers* © Sue Jennings 2019

87 Dragons 2

⊙ Groups
Individuals may also create their own collage ideas.

Resources

Collage materials such as sequins and fabrics, white glue; coloured pens, one very large piece of card or thick paper.

Description

Dragons frequently occupy a central place in mythology, demonstrating that they represent something important to the human psyche.

Learning Outcomes

- A wider knowledge of dragon imagery
- Understanding ancient truths surrounding dragons
- Being able to externalise the 'dragons' inside us
- Coming to terms with fear and anxiety

Activities

- Explore the idea of the whole group creating a dragon.
- Using a large piece of paper, encourage somebody to draw an outline of a dragon.
- Group members fill in the outline with different dragon features.
- Using coloured pens, link up all the aspects of the dragon drawing.

Attachment Relevance

Group relationships help to overcome anxiety and fear of others, as teenagers unite to create a single image.

This page may be photocopied for instructional use only. *Working with Attachment Difficulties in Teenagers* © Sue Jennings 2019

88 Dragons 3

⊙ Individuals & groups

Resources

Coloured pens/pencils, scissors; Worksheet 15, 'The Dragon Mask', for each person.

Description

Moving on from the picture of the dragon in Activity 87 to a representation of a dragon's head used as a mask.

Learning Outcomes

- Working in the three dimensions
- Following clear instructions
- Satisfaction at completion
- Accepting a 'good enough' piece of art

Activities

- Using the worksheet, colour the dragon mask.
- Use the picture of the mask to prompt a dragon story.
- Cut out the mask.
- Speak the story in role, as the dragon.

Attachment Relevance

Developing confidence to be in a self-directed role.

P This page may be photocopied for instructional use only. *Working with Attachment Difficulties in Teenagers* © Sue Jennings 2019

89 Dragons 4

⊙ Individuals & groups

Resources

Card (three pieces per person), poster paint and brushes.

Description

This activity explores contrasting ideas about dragons and communicated similarities and differences.

Learning Outcomes

- Encourages flexibility
- Developing shape and colour
- Relates image to story
- Associates word and picture

Activities

- Each person has three pieces of card.
- Paint three contrasting dragon images.
- Explore the dominant feature, such as eyes or nostrils or claws.
- Think of a story to link the three dragons.

Attachment Relevance

Developing flexible relationships between art, image and others.

This page may be photocopied for instructional use only. *Working with Attachment Difficulties in Teenagers* © Sue Jennings 2019

90 Dragons 5

⊙ Groups

Resources

Flexible card and strong stapler, scissors, pencils and poster paint, paint brushes; a large piece of cloth to paint on.

Description

This is a collaborative exercise, during which members of the whole group jointly create one dragon.

Learning Outcomes

- Cooperation between individuals
- Acceptance of others' ideas
- Allowing other people to lead
- Physically coordinating together

Activities

- Using the card, draw the pieces to make a three-dimensional dragon mask, then paint it, cut it out and assemble it with the stapler.
- Use the cloth as the body of the dragon.
- Paint its scales and skin.
- Experiment with everyone being a part of the dragon, taking it in turns to carry the dragon's head in front.

Attachment Relevance

The synthesis of these activities is manifested in peer attachment within the group, creating images and movement together.

This page may be photocopied for instructional use only. *Working with Attachment Difficulties in Teenagers* © Sue Jennings 2019

Part 4
Integrated Themes: Weaving the Threads

This shorter section brings together several themes in one series of activities, in order for participants to feel a sense of wholeness. Many teenagers will have become one-dimensional in their perceptions, as if it is too much to hold on to the whole of life. These sessions, which accommodate those who enjoy being 'larger than life' as well as those who prefer to be 'in miniature', are designed to include techniques from earlier sections of the book. However, the techniques are combined, rather than sequenced, and provide opportunities for choices of media.

For example, the dragon-making exercise (Activity 90, 'Dragon 5') is a collaborative technique that encourages group members to work together. In the following integrated themes the dragon is placed within the context of a story, a culture and events. It is working in a multi-dimensional structure where people can play contrasting roles and eat celebratory food.

Additionally, the story of the Dragon Boat Festival supplies the opportunity to explore loss and mourning, as well as life and celebration. The idea of miniature theatres allows participants to create performed narratives that may be from the dragon boat story, or may be personal.

The Dragon Boat Festival also provides an opportunity for the exploration of a story (see Story Sheet 2) within a cultural context. Participants have the opportunity to make dragon boats from cardboard (Activity 91) and then race them (Activity 92), followed by eating celebratory food (Activity 93). Then there are the press interviews and photographs that follow any cultural celebration (Activity 94). The death of the Chinese poet Qu Yuan is explored (Activity 95), as well as the poetry he wrote (Activity 96). The story of a poet who lived is created (Activity 97) and a play is made from the story (Activity 98). A miniature story theatre is formed (Activity 99) and the story is performed (Activity 100). Allow photographs to be taken if possible.

91 Dragon Boats

⊙ Groups

Resources

Light weight card, scissors, sticky tape, white glue, staplers, coloured pens or acrylic paints and paintbrushes, pictures of dragon boats (there are plenty on Google Images); Story Sheet 2, 'The Dragon Boat Festival', for each person.

Description

Dragon boats can be created in pairs from card and coloured with individual symbols. Use the images you collect to inspire ideas! Allow photographs to be taken if possible.

Learning Outcomes

- Collaboration with a partner
- Negotiation on creative decisions
- Resolution of structure
- Expansion of ideas

Activities

- Tell the story of the Dragon Boat Race given on the story sheet.
- Share images of dragon boats from Google Images.
- In pairs create a dragon boat from card, tape and staples.
- Negotiate colours and symbols and share boats together.

Attachment Relevance

Encouraging creativity through collaboration.

This page may be photocopied for instructional use only. *Working with Attachment Difficulties in Teenagers* © Sue Jennings 2019

92 The Dragon Boat Race

⦿ Groups

Resources

Large blue cloth or blue paper to represent the water; bamboo sticks with masking tape over the ends for safety, boats made in Activity 91, rice, a drum and another 'chime' instrument for improvised Chinese-sounding music to introduce and end the race; Story Sheet 2, 'The Dragon Boat Festival'.

Description

Using a large blue cloth or blue paper, people 'race' their boats over the water, remembering at the same time that they are actually looking for the body of the poet (see Story Sheet 2). Rice is sprinkled for the fish to eat, just as in the story. The race is preceded by Chinese music and a drumbeat to start. More music at the end of the race, with a final drumbeat. Allow photographs to be taken, if possible.

Learning Outcomes

- Exploring 'safe' competition
- Experiencing that it is fine to lose sometimes
- Learning to hold two concepts in mind at the same time (racing and searching)
- Encouraging the development of symbols in art and expression

Activities

- Practise some sounds on the instruments and agree that a single drumbeat starts the race.
- Group people around the water and agree which pair will race first; sprinkle some rice for the fish (see story sheet).
- Pairs propel their boats with the bamboo stick – thwacking is not allowed!
- At the same time they are looking for the poet in the water.

Attachment Relevance

The race enables sequencing and collaboration, with several themes running parallel.

This page may be photocopied for instructional use only. *Working with Attachment Difficulties in Teenagers* © Sue Jennings 2019

93 Dragon Boat Celebration

⊙ Groups

Resources

Recipe for *Zongzi* (see Appendix 2, 'Recipes: Celebratory Food'), ingredients, including fillings; access to a cooking ring (gas or electric), cooking utensils and saucepan. Table and chairs, blue tablecloth, candles or electric tea-lights, plates and spoons (real rather than plastic, if possible); dragon boats made in Activity 91; Story Sheet 2, 'The Dragon Boat Festival'.

Description

Cooking and enjoying a celebratory meal can be a session on its own, or form part of Activity 92. The recipe for sticky rice balls (*Zongzi*) is in Appendix 2, 'Recipes: Celebratory Food', and takes roughly 30 minutes to make. A filling is put in the middle of the balls as they are shaped. The balls were wrapped in bamboo or corn leaves, however, I suggest rice paper or greaseproof paper is used for simplicity. The food is eaten as a celebration, while the story is read. Allow photographs to be taken, if possible.

Learning Outcomes

- Incorporating various activities into one event
- Taking turns and waiting
- Experiencing new food within a celebration
- Affirmation of the experiences in Activities 91 & 92

Activities

- Everyone helps to rinse the rice, and then places it in saucepan, covered in water, to cook.
- Everyone shares the task of preparing the table with cloth, model boats, candles, plates, spoons.
- A rice ball is placed on each plate, wrapped in rice paper or greaseproof paper.
- Everyone gives their portion to someone else, and someone reads the story while the rice is eaten.

Attachment Relevance

The group are sharing a nurturing experience of cooking and preparing food together, and then offering it to others.

This page may be photocopied for instructional use only. *Working with Attachment Difficulties in Teenagers* © Sue Jennings 2019

94 Dragon Boat Press Reports & Photographs

⊙ Groups

Resources

Any photos taken during the previous sessions, A4 & A2 paper, rulers and pencils, rubbers (reluctantly), coloured pens, scissors, whiteboard and markers.

Description

Participants are encouraged to reflect on the previous activities (boat-making, racing, celebration of food) and discuss how they could be written up in a newspaper, together with the photographs. Working in groups of three or four, each group creates a news sheet.

Learning Outcomes

- Improving literacy
- Connecting experience with written and visual imagery
- Learning control over stories and their expression
- Discovering 'less is more'

Activities

- Working in groups of three or four at separate tables, brainstorm ideas together and write them on the whiteboard.
- Share the way that a newspaper can report on an event from a different perspective.
- Each group designs their own news sheet, with short written descriptions in 'boxes' and photos.
- Share the finished news sheets, making sure everyone's efforts are affirmed.

Attachment Relevance

Collaboration with peers creates attachment and affirmation of each other's creative ideas and objects.

This page may be photocopied for instructional use only. *Working with Attachment Difficulties in Teenagers* © Sue Jennings 2019

95 Reflecting on the Poet who Died

⊙ Individuals & groups

Note Use of Activities 95 & 96 will depend on recent experiences of loss and bereavement within the group and how well group members are dealing with what has happened. However, working with a 'distanced' example of death by suicide can help young people address their complex feeling.

Resources

Paper, coloured pens and pencils, tissue paper and glue; Story Sheet 2, 'The Dragon Boat Festival'.

Description

This session is a time for reflection, while the story of the Dragon Boat Festival is read again and members of the group are invited to consider the loss of the young poet and its implications.

Learning Outcomes

- Expressing feelings about loss and death
- Sharing reflections about suicide
- Contributing ideas about the acknowledgement of death
- Allowing deeper feelings to be shared

Activities

- Read the story, or suggest someone or several people in the group read it out loud.
- Share thoughts and feelings about the death and how it is celebrated.
- Invite group members to express their feelings through the art materials.
- Share pictures and images

Attachment Relevance

Acknowledging loss is part of the attachment process.

This page may be photocopied for instructional use only. *Working with Attachment Difficulties in Teenagers* © Sue Jennings 2019

96 Poetry for the Poet who Died

⊙ Individuals & groups

Note Decisions on the use of Activities 95 & 96 will depend on recent experiences of loss and bereavement within the group and how well group members are dealing with what has happened. However, working with a 'distanced' example of death by suicide can help young people address their complex feeling.

Resources

Your own choice of poems to share with the group (mine would be examples from Dylan Thomas and Shakespeare's Sonnets, also the beautiful lines in Shakespeare's *Cymbeline* (Act IV, scene ii), which start, 'Fear no more the heat o' the sun …'); a rhyming dictionary, paper, pens, newspapers (for cutting out words), glue, scissors.

Description

This workshop encourages young people to express their feelings through simple poetry and leads to an understanding of the importance of poetry.

Learning Outcomes

- Building confidence through writing achievement
- Giving form to feelings
- Acknowledging the importance of feelings and loss and death
- Understanding the importance of poetry

Activities

- Share one or two of your choice of poems and reflect on the images and themes.
- Play with words on paper that might be included in a poem (use the rhyming dictionary).
- Create your own poem by writing words or cutting out newspaper words.
- Decorate the poem and share with the group.

Attachment Relevance

Working with poetry enables the expression of feelings.

This page may be photocopied for instructional use only. *Working with Attachment Difficulties in Teenagers* © Sue Jennings 2019

97 Story of a Poet who Lived

⊙ Groups

Resources

Paper, pencils and pens.

Description

The focus is on a poet (or author, or other people chosen by the group), someone who either exists or is imagined: this person's story is written.

Learning Outcomes

- Creating narrative structure
- Giving form to ideas
- Practising sequencing
- Developing resolutions

Activities

- Discuss the interest in a person's story.
- Is our interest in their achievements or their behaviour?
- Structure ideas in small groups to create a story.
- Write and share the story.

Attachment Relevance

Creating attachments, or recognising the lack of them, through the story.

This page may be photocopied for instructional use only. *Working with Attachment Difficulties in Teenagers* © Sue Jennings 2019

98 Making a Play from the Story

⊙ Groups

Resources

Paper and pens.

Description

Having created stories, the group members look at how stories become plays or films, then choose stories created in Activity 98 to transform into plays.

Learning Outcomes

- Learning about scripts for performance
- Describing roles and characters
- Improving observations and detail
- Encouraging interest in theatre and plays

Activities

- Discuss dramas, live or on TV, that group members have seen.
- How does a story become a play?
- Work in groups of two or three to make a play from the stories.
- Read the play out to others.

Attachment Relevance

Structuring experience into narrative allows people to live in their own attachment.

This page may be photocopied for instructional use only. *Working with Attachment Difficulties in Teenagers* © Sue Jennings 2019

99 Creating a Story Theatre

⊙ Individuals & groups

Note The creation of the Story Theatre will take more than one session and it is important that participants are not rushed, particularly since some fiddly work is involved and achievement is very important.

Resources

One shoe box per person (suitcase boxes are also obtainable from craft shops); magazines (to create the audience), pipe-cleaners or similar, wool (for covering pipe cleaners), glue, craft wood (for making scenery/props), cardboard, scraps of material, scissors for everyone, paints.

Description

A Story Theatre is a small theatre created out of a shoe box, or similar. Characters and props can be added and stories enacted.

Learning Outcomes

- Sense of achievement in creating a finished product
- Learning of accumulation process, from story to theatre
- Opportunity to enact a story as a play
- Encouragement of theatre as a learning medium

Activities

- Show how the box can be placed on its long side on the upside-down lid, so that the lid becomes a stage and the box is where the audience sit to watch.
- Cut out people from magazines and stick them inside the box, in front of the 'stage' created by the lid. This is the audience.
- Decide on props and make them, using craft wood, cardboard and material.
- Decide on the characters needed for the play, creating them with craft wood, cardboard, pipe-cleaners and material (or use miniature dolls, if available).

Attachment Relevance

The affirmation from this creativity is very important for people with attachment difficulties.

This page may be photocopied for instructional use only. *Working with Attachment Difficulties in Teenagers* © Sue Jennings 2019

(100) Performing in the Story Theatre

⊙ Individuals & groups

Please Note It is important that there is time for discussion and presentation of Certificates of Achievement (see Worksheet 16). You may decide to have a further session for processing and closure. Group members will also wish to see and keep the photos.

Resources

Story Theatres, props and characters from Activity 99; camera or phone.

Description

When group members have completed their Story Theatre, it is time to perform the plays they have created from the stories. Everyone needs the opportunity to perform their play.

Learning Outcomes

- Integrating all the learning (which is a function of theatre)
- Experiencing three-dimensional creativity
- Transforming story into theatre
- Improving performance confidence

Activities

- Everyone has time to practise/rehearse their story.
- Group members take it in turns to present their play.
- Take pictures of their theatre and performance.
- Spend time discussing the project as a whole, as well as this session.

Attachment Relevance

All of the skills learned in this programme are those experienced in a healthy attachment relationship.

This page may be photocopied for instructional use only. *Working with Attachment Difficulties in Teenagers* © Sue Jennings 2019

Worksheets & Story Sheets

Worksheets

Story Sheets

1 This is My Brain 1

Activity: 40

Colour the reptilian part of the brain.

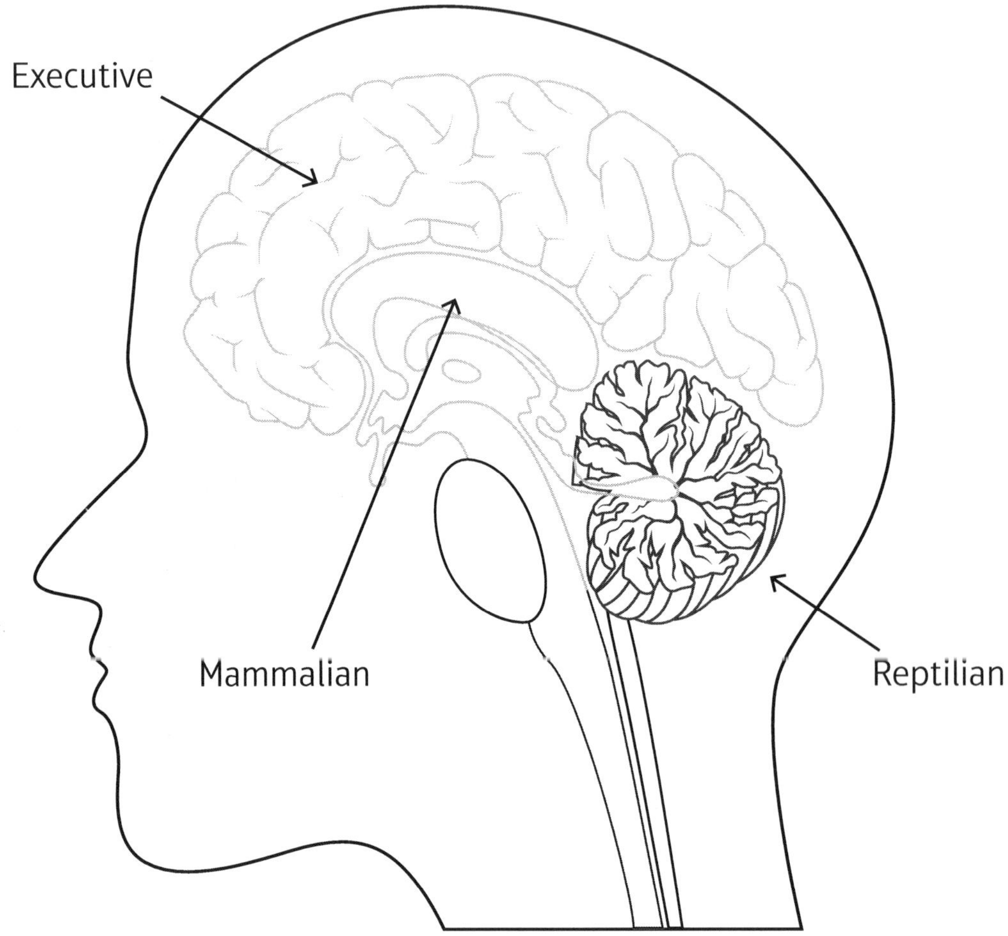

Draw a reptile and write or draw its qualities.

This page may be photocopied for instructional use only. *Working with Attachment Difficulties in Teenagers* © Sue Jennings 2019

2 This is My Brain 2

Activity: 41

Colour the mammalian part of the brain.

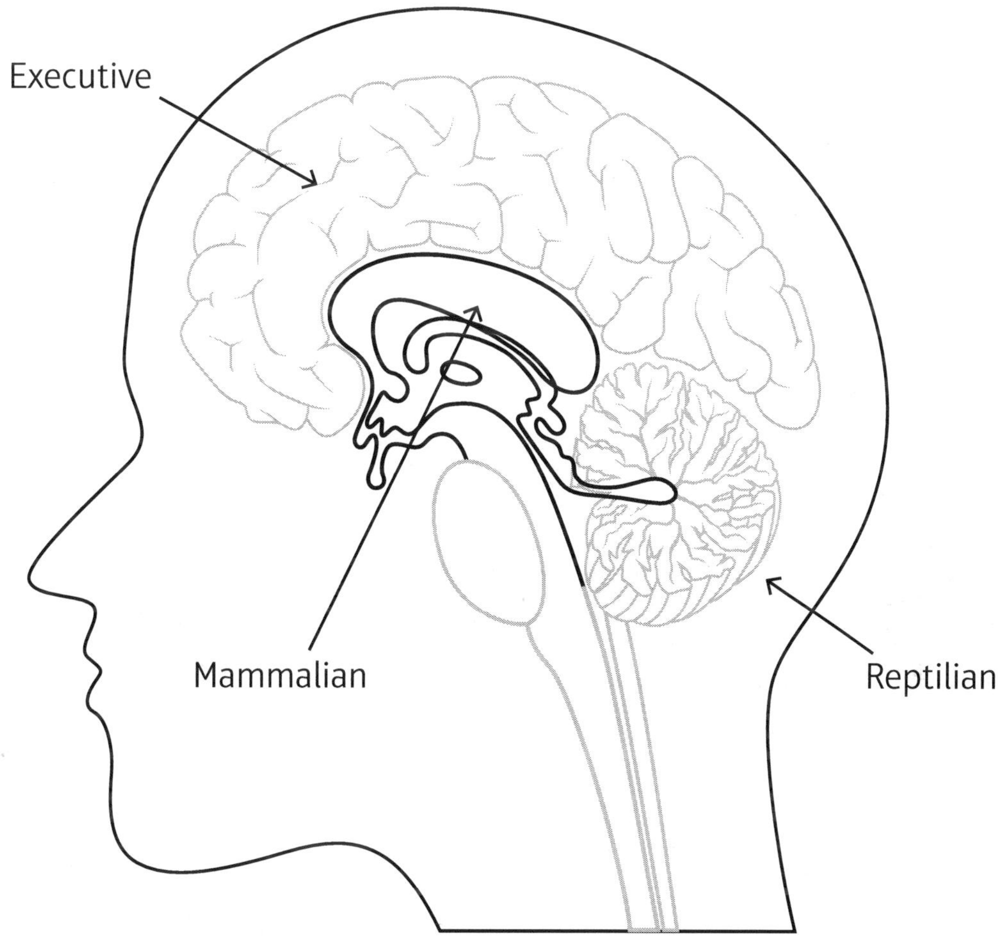

Draw a mammal and write or draw its qualities.

This page may be photocopied for instructional use only. *Working with Attachment Difficulties in Teenagers* © Sue Jennings 2019

3 This is My Brain 3

Activity: 42

Colour the executive function part of the brain.

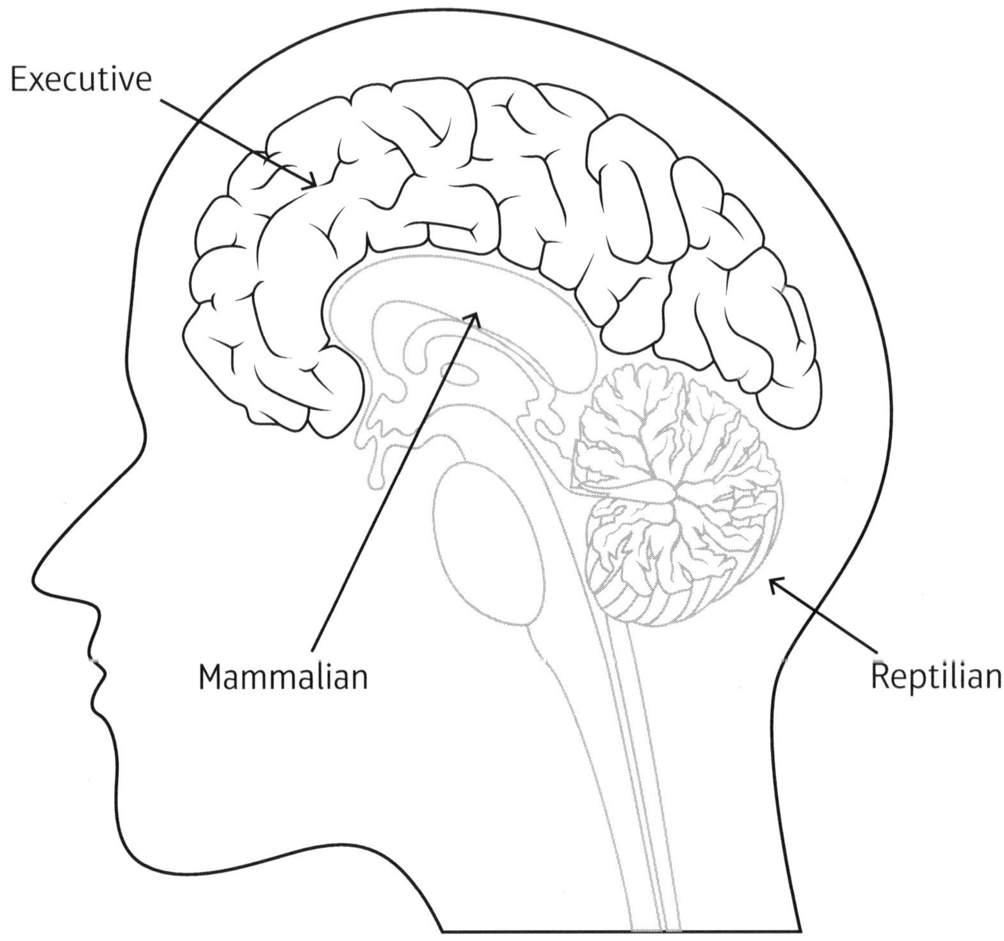

Draw a teenager, male or female, and write and draw their qualities.

This page may be photocopied for instructional use only. *Working with Attachment Difficulties in Teenagers* © Sue Jennings 2019

4 Inside My Head

Activity: 44

Write or draw, and colour the thoughts and feelings that are 'inside your head'.

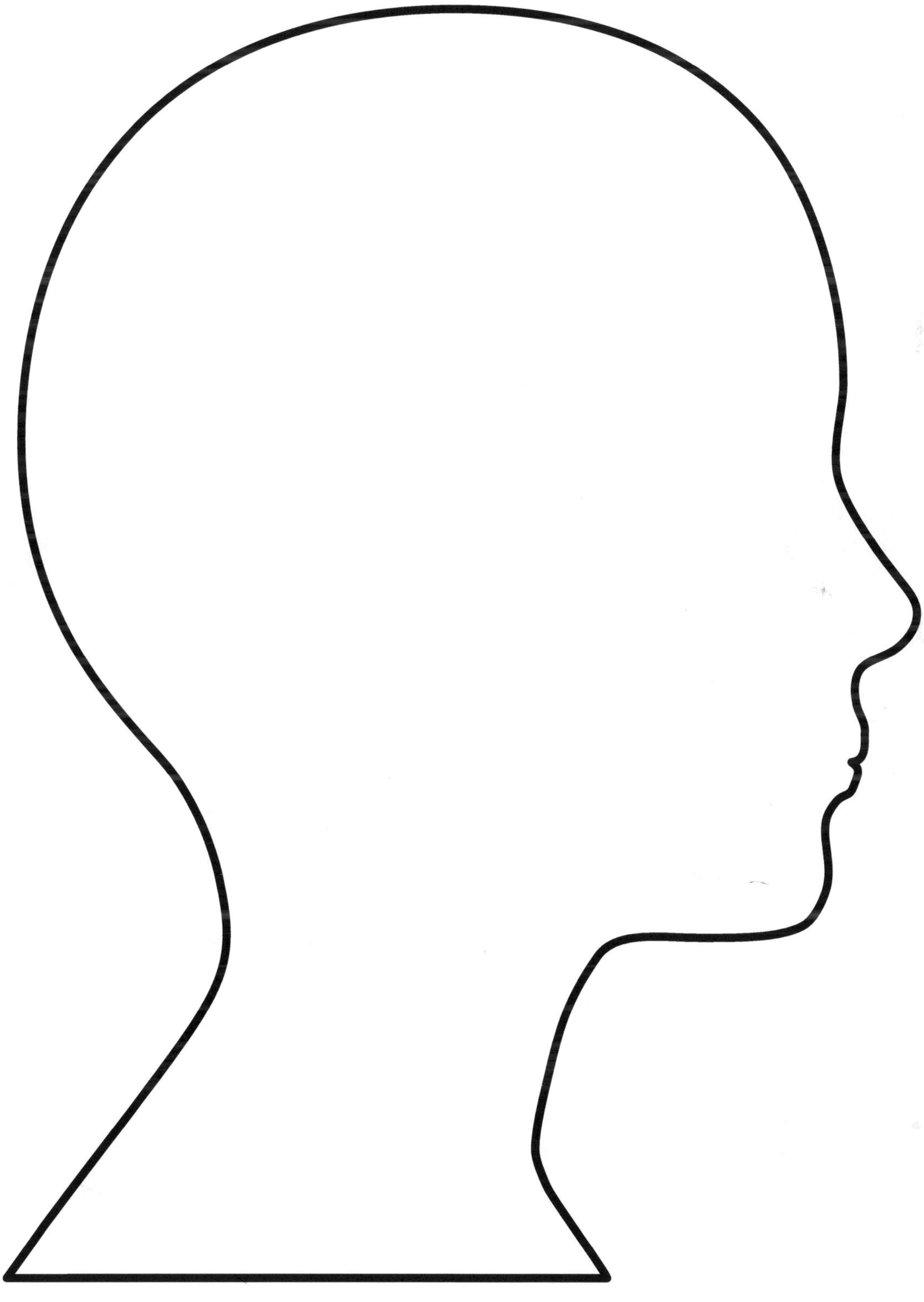

This page may be photocopied for instructional use only. *Working with Attachment Difficulties in Teenagers* © Sue Jennings 2019

5 Inside Your Head

Activity: 45

Write or draw, and colour the thoughts and feelings that you think are inside someone else's head.

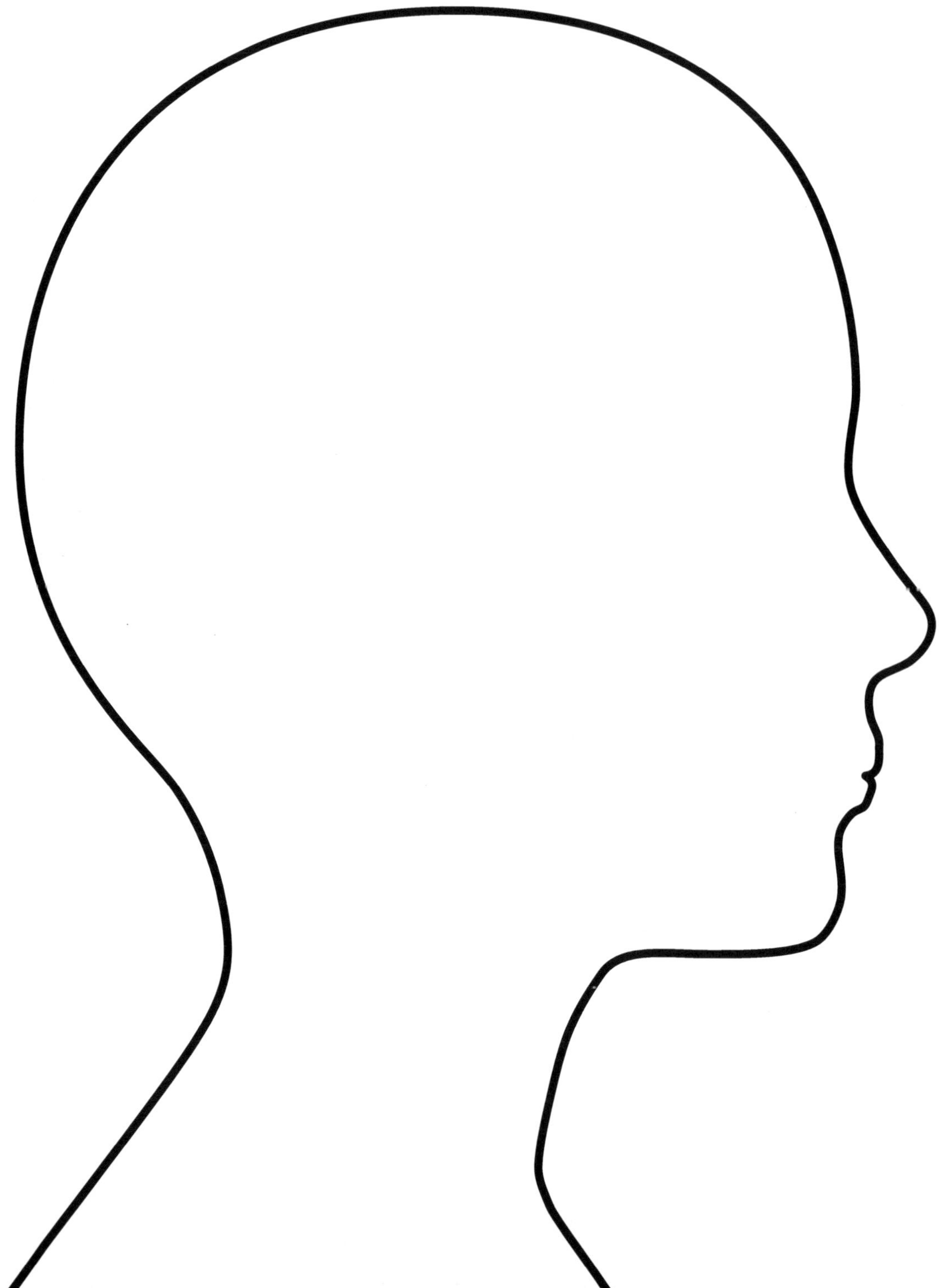

This page may be photocopied for instructional use only. *Working with Attachment Difficulties in Teenagers* © Sue Jennings 2019

6 Who do I Admire?

Activity: 46

Describe in words or pictures, the qualities that you admire in another person.

How they dress: ______________________

____

____

____

Their personality: ______________________

____

____

____

Their skills: ______________________

____

____

____

The way they speak: ______________________

____

____

____

Other qualities: ______________________

____

____

____

Worksheet 6

This page may be photocopied for instructional use only. *Working with Attachment Difficulties in Teenagers* © Sue Jennings 2019

7 Shakespeare Role-Play: Girlfriends

Activity: 76

A brief scene from Shakespeare's *A Midsummer Night's Dream* (Act I: scene i) illustrates the reality of teenage friendships. In this extract Hermia and Helena are arguing over the same potential boyfriend. Hermia's father wishes her to marry Demetrius, whereas she wants to marry Lysander. Helena wants to marry Demetrius and complains how Hermia is more attractive to him.

Would they wear hats or scarves? Carry a bag or tote?

> Hermia: I frown upon him, yet he loves me still.
>
> Helena: Oh, that your frowns would teach my smiles such skill!
>
> Hermia: I give him curses, yet he gives me love.
>
> Helena: Oh, that my prayers could such affection move!
>
> Hermia: The more I hate, the more he follows me.
>
> Helena: The more I love, the more he hateth me.
>
> Hermia: His folly, Helena, is no fault of mine.
>
> Helena: None, but your beauty. Would that fault were mine!

Read the text in pairs, swapping roles and using different voices and gestures; how does it feel when you speak the words very quickly and then very slowly? Does it make a difference if the two people look at each other? Try the scene with one person looking away. Remember that Helena and Hermia are best friends.

How must it feel when the boy you want to go out with only pays attention to someone else? How can this be expressed in the role-play? What do you think Helena writes in her diary?

This page may be photocopied for instructional use only. *Working with Attachment Difficulties in Teenagers* © Sue Jennings 2019

8 Shakespeare Role-Play: Father & Daughter

Activity: 77

In this brief scene from *Romeo and Juliet* (Act III, scene v) between Juliet and her mother and her father, he has lost his temper, because she won't do his bidding. He is trying to force her to marry Paris, but Juliet is in love with Romeo. Romeo is in hiding because he has killed Juliet's brother, Tybalt; Tybalt had killed Mercutio a close friend of Romeo. Juliet is trying to delay everything by saying she needs more time to mourn the death of her brother. Her father loses patience when she tells him that, although she is thankful for the arrangements he has made on her behalf, she cannot be proud to marry Paris.

What props might be useful?

Juliet [to her mother]: I wonder at this haste, that I must wed

Ere he, that should be husband, comes to woo.

I pray you tell my lord and father, madam,

I will not marry yet …

Father: … Mistress minion you,

Thank me no thankings, nor proud me no prouds,

But fettle your fine joints 'gainst Thursday next

To go with Paris to Saint Peter's Church,

Or I will drag thee on a hurdle thither …

Read the text in pairs, swapping roles and using different voices and gestures: how does it feel when you speak the words very quietly and then very loudly? Does it make a difference if the two people look at each other? Try the scene with one person looking away, or with Juliet crouching and her father towering over her.

How must it feel when your lover has killed your brother in a street brawl? What are the real choices that Juliet has to make?

This page may be photocopied for instructional use only. *Working with Attachment Difficulties in Teenagers* © Sue Jennings 2019

9 Shakespeare Role-Play: King & Helper

Activity: 78

In this scene from *A Midsummer Night's Dream* (Act III, scene ii) between Oberon and Puck, it turns out that Puck has put the love-juice (a magical potion that causes people to fall in love with the first person or creature they see when they awake) on the eyes of the wrong man. So a true lover has woken up and fallen in love with someone else! Oberon is angry and sends Puck off to find Helena so he can put things right!

Do they need a simple costume? A hat or a cloak?

Oberon: What hast thou done? Thou hast mistaken quite,
And laid the love juice on some true love's sight.
Of thy misprision must perforce ensue
Some true love turned, and not a false turned true.
Puck: Then fate o'errules that, one man holding troth
A million fail, confounding oath on oath.
Oberon: About the wood go swifter than the wind,
And Helena of Athens look thou find –
… By some illusion see thou bring her here.
I'll charm his eyes against she do appear.
Puck: I go, I go. Look how I go,
Swifter than arrow from the Tartar's bow.

Read the text in pairs, swapping roles and using different voices and gestures. How does it feel when you speak the words in a very clipped way, and then very loudly? Does it make a difference if the two people look at each other? Try it with one person looking away. Is Puck really sorry he has made a mistake? The last line implies that he goes very quickly – try the scene with him doing the opposite, and annoying Oberon even more!

How must it feel when you have done the wrong thing? Think of a time when you have made a mistake and a parent or teacher is very angry.

This page may be photocopied for instructional use only. *Working with Attachment Difficulties in Teenagers* © Sue Jennings 2019

10 Shakespeare Role-Play: Chorus (*Henry V*)

Activity: 79

This is a short extract from the speech given by the Chorus who open *Henry V* (Act I, Prologue). The chorus sets the theme for the play of a 'larger than life' story of heroics, loss, sadness and romance. It also uses Shakespeare's favourite metaphor for the theatre itself: 'A kingdom for a stage …'

Are props needed?

Chorus: O for a muse of fire, that would ascend
The brightest heaven of invention,
A kingdom for a stage, princes to act
And monarchs to behold the swelling scene!
Then should the warlike Harry, like himself,
Assume the port of Mars; and at his heels,
Leash'd in like hounds, should famine, sword and fire
Crouch for employment.

Read the text in pairs, swapping roles and using different voices and gestures. How does it feel when you speak the words in a powerful way and then in a thoughtful way? In a group experiment with each person reading only one line: does it make more sense? Does it deepen your understanding?

Think about when you have had to make a speech to inspire people. Read the speech again, believing that it will persuade others to listen to and believe what you are saying.

This page may be photocopied for instructional use only. *Working with Attachment Difficulties in Teenagers* © Sue Jennings 2019

11 Shakespeare Role-Play: Lovers

Activity: 80

These two extracts are from *Twelfth Night* (Act I, scenes i & v): the two speeches by Orsino and Viola illustrate the power of imagery when talking of love. In the play the two characters are not speaking to each other about their love, but to someone else. Orsino is in love with Olivia, who uses the excuse of mourning the death of her father to avoid engaging with him. Viola, who is disguised as a boy, is in love with Orsino, but is acting as a messenger between Olivia and Orsino. Just to complicate matters, Olivia, believing Viola to be a boy, falls in love with 'him'!

Will you use costumes or other props?

Orsino: If music be the food of love, play on;
Give me excess of it that, surfeiting,
The appetite may sicken and so die.
That strain again, it had a dying fall;
O it came o'er my ear like the sweet sound
That breathes upon a bank of violets,
Stealing and giving odour. Act I, scene i

Viola: Make me a willow cabin at your gate,
And call upon my soul within the house,
Write loyal cantons of contemnèd love
And sing them loud even in the dead of night; Act I, scene v

Remember that this is not a dialogue between these two characters, however, read the speeches in pairs, using different voices and gestures. How does it feel when you speak the words desperately, or lovingly, or with humour? Imagine these are the words of a pop song, who would be singing it? Then swap roles.

How must it feel when you love someone and they do not reciprocate? Note that Olivia uses the same excuse that Juliet does (mourning deaths of father or brother).

This page may be photocopied for instructional use only. *Working with Attachment Difficulties in Teenagers* © Sue Jennings 2019

12 Rapunzel 1

Activity: 84

This is the tower in the woods:

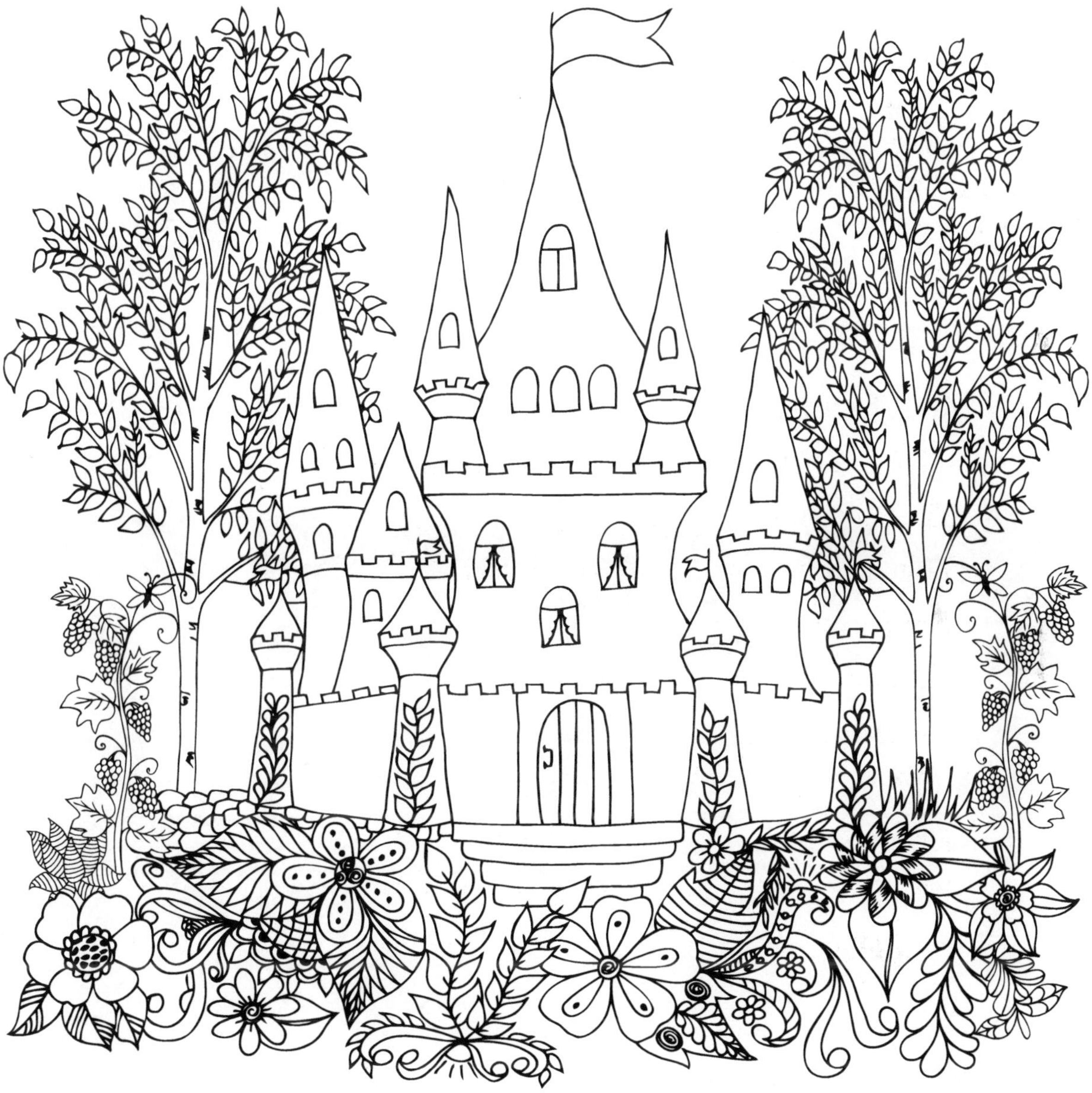

Use the image provided or draw your own of the woods and the tower where Rapunzel was imprisoned and colour it in.

This page may be photocopied for instructional use only. *Working with Attachment Difficulties in Teenagers* © Sue Jennings 2019

13 Rapunzel 2

Activity: 84

The Rapunzel flower is called *Campanula rapunculus*, or rampion bellflower.

The flower of the Rapunzel plant is very simple and beautiful: it is white, tinged palest purple. The leaves of the plant are eaten as a vegetable, like spinach, and the roots can be cooked too, like parsnips.

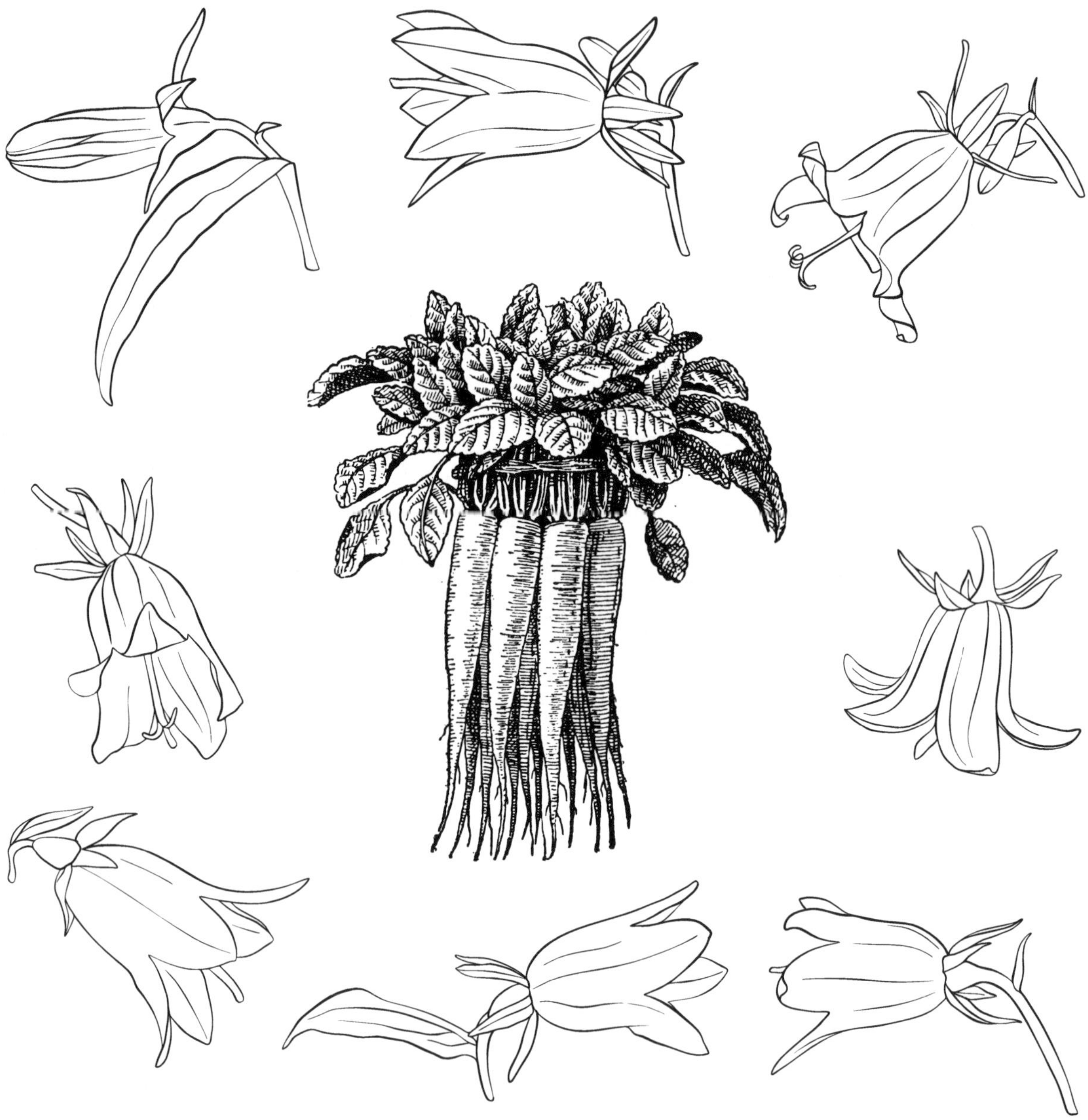

Colour the flower, leaves and roots.

Why do you think the authors of the story, the Brothers Grimm, choose this name for their heroine?

This page may be photocopied for instructional use only. *Working with Attachment Difficulties in Teenagers* © Sue Jennings 2019

14 Rapunzel 3

Activity: 84

There is a Disney version of the Rapunzel story, in which she has a chameleon friend and together they wonder what the world beyond the tower is like.

Draw your own picture of Rapunzel and give her a friend of your own choosing.

Draw or write down things that they might imagine and talk about in the big world.

This page may be photocopied for instructional use only. *Working with Attachment Difficulties in Teenagers* © Sue Jennings 2019

15 The Dragon Mask

Activity: 88

Colour the dragon's head in your choice of colours.

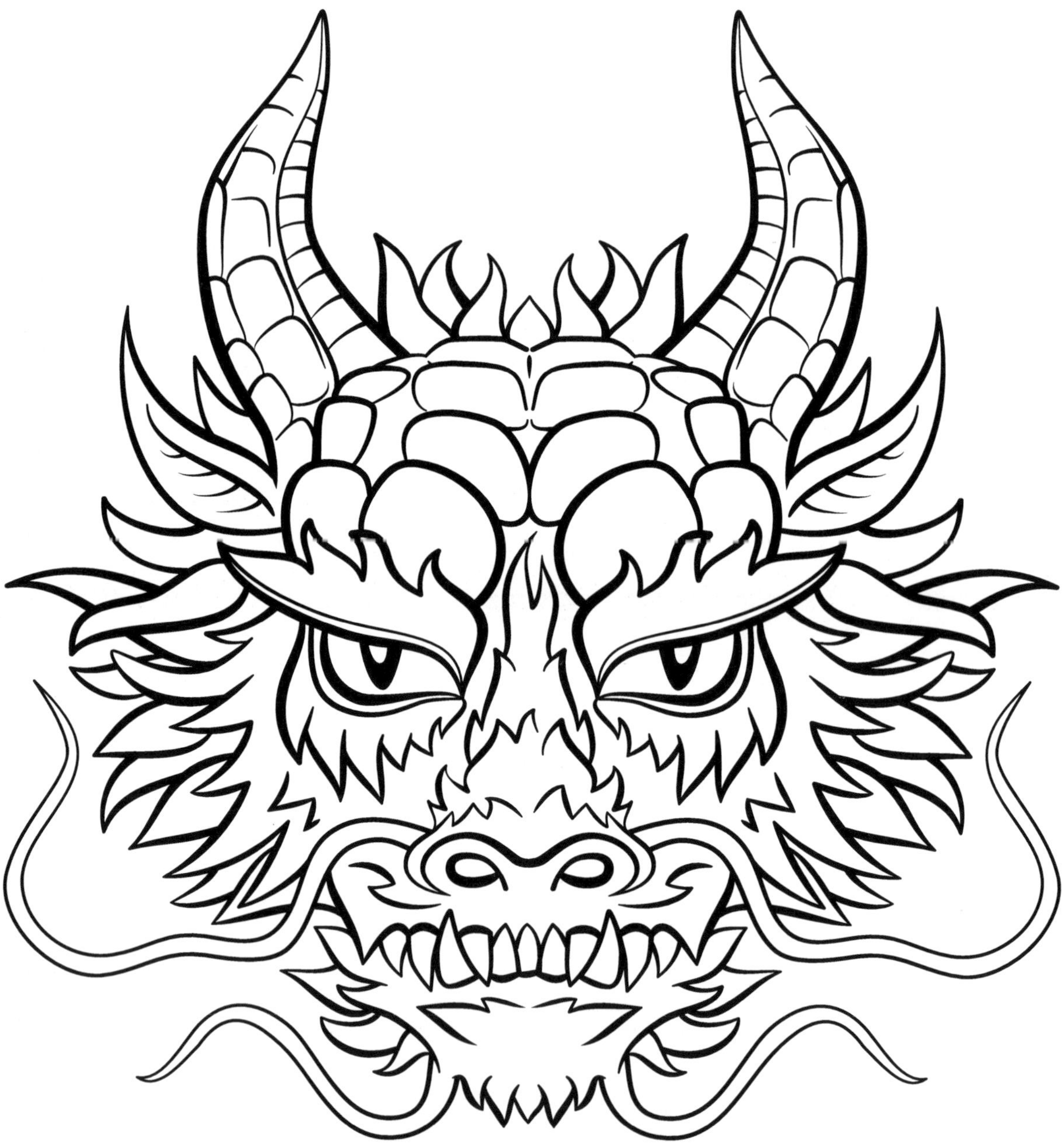

This page may be photocopied for instructional use only. *Working with Attachment Difficulties in Teenagers* © Sue Jennings 2019

16 Certificate of Achievement

Activity: 100

CERTIFICATE

awarded to

____

for attending this

Course

and showing changes in

1 ______________________________________

2 ______________________________________

3 ______________________________________

Signed ________________________

Project Leader

Date ________________________

This page may be photocopied for instructional use only. *Working with Attachment Difficulties in Teenagers* © Sue Jennings 2019

S1 The Story of Rapunzel

Activity: 84

Once upon a time a man and woman longed to have a child. After many years, the wife conceived and they were both very happy. However, the wife became very ill and slowly became weaker and weaker.

The husband grew desperate: he could think of nothing to help her. At last, feeling very frightened, he decided to go into the garden of the witch next door and pick one of her herbs that were used for medicine.

Unfortunately the witch saw him and said he would be cursed, but he begged and pleaded, and eventually she said that he could have the herb, but that they must give the child to the witch once she was 10 years old.

Ten years after the child's birth, the witch took her and locked her in a tall tower in the forest with no entrance. The child was named Rapunzel, after the Rapunzel flower that had made her mother well: she was very beautiful and had very long hair. The witch would arrive with food and call out, 'Rapunzel, let down your hair', and the witch would climb up her hair into the tower. Rapunzel was very sad and lonely and would sing and cry at her window.

As she grew older, it happened that a prince was riding by and saw this beautiful young woman at her window. As the witch approached, the prince hid and so he heard the witch call out to Rapunzel to let down her hair. The next day the prince returned and called out to her let down her hair, which she did. They fell deeply in love and the prince visited Rapunzel every night.

Page 1 of 2

This page may be photocopied for instructional use only. *Working with Attachment Difficulties in Teenagers* © Sue Jennings 2019

S1 The Story of Rapunzel

Activity: 84

However, one evening the witch arrived and found the prince in the tower. She was very angry and pushed him out of the window into a thorn bush where he was blinded. She banished Rapunzel to the desert.

The prince was wandering through the lands, wondering what had happened to this beautiful woman. One day he could hear Rapunzel singing and he moved in the direction of her voice. She saw him and hugged him very tight, crying tears of joy. As the tears ran down the prince's face, his sight was restored. He took Rapunzel back to his kingdom and they were very happy together.

You can discuss this story or even dramatise it, if you wish. Worksheets 12, 13 and 14 give you more activities and opportunities to reflect on the Rapunzel story.

This page may be photocopied for instructional use only. *Working with Attachment Difficulties in Teenagers* © Sue Jennings 2019

S2 The Dragon Boat Festival

Activities: 91, 92, 93, 95

Dragon Boat Festival (known as the 'Duanwu Festival' in China) is celebrated on the fifth day of the fifth month of the Chinese calendar

It commemorates the life and death of poet Qu Yuan, who drowned himself in the Miluo River. Qu Yuan was a famous Chinese scholar who was exiled, following accusations by envious court officials. He wrote many poems expressing his anger and sorrow at what had happened and then drowned himself. Many people believed he was a good person, accused unjustly, and they frantically took to their boats to try and save him. They even dropped lumps of rice into the river to stop the fish eating his body. But Qu Yuan's body was never found.

The Festival commemorates this frantic search with dragon boat races and every family eats *Zongzi* during the Festival, a sticky rice dumpling wrapped in bamboo leaves.

There are many other ways that this Festival is celebrated, especially in relation to health and healing: plants (mugwort) are hung on doors to prevent disease, perfumed sachets are carried, and water drawn at midday is said to have healing properties.

A dragon boat is a paddle boat that can have up to 80 rowers, depending on size. The front is shaped like an open-mouthed dragon and the back has a tail. After the boats are built, the dragon's eyes are finally painted in a sacred ceremony that symbolises 'bringing the boat to life'.

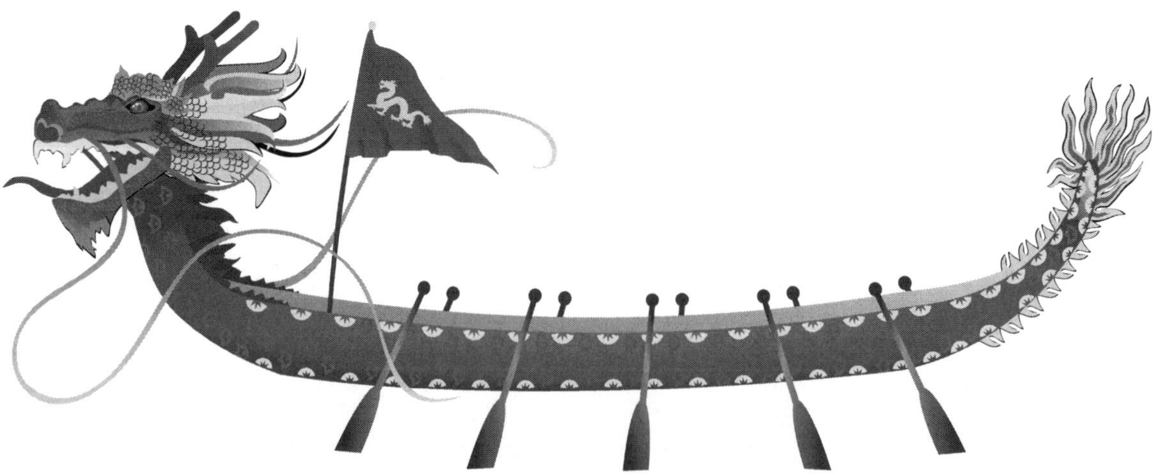

The Dragon Boat Festival is one of UNESCO's 'Intangible Cultural Heritage Items'.

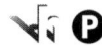

This page may be photocopied for instructional use only. *Working with Attachment Difficulties in School-Aged Children* © Sue Jennings 2018

Appendix 1
Drama Games & Warm Ups

Using the Directory of Games & Warm-Ups

These exercises vary from a very simple walk to a more complex game. They are ideal as an introduction to 'action learning' and provide a basis for confidence-building. Their most important function is to 'warm-up' – to focus energy. When choosing warm-ups, it is important that they are linked to the activities in the group and not chosen at random. A warm-up is just that, it warms up the body and the brain, ready for creative activity.

I usually start with physical warm-ups, because often there is surplus energy that needs to be focused and then transformed. My approach does not work with angry expression for its own sake, such as smashing old china or breaking bricks: I use physical energy that expresses angry energy and then turns it into something else.

For example, a physical game of throwing and catching the soft ball focuses scattered energy and allows it to become collaborative energy. A jog around the park encourages a 'feel good' factor and prepares group members for focussed group work. In all warm-ups it is important to remember awareness of breathing, whether to create energy or to bring about relaxation.

1 Breathing & voice 1

Exercises to be repeated 3 or 4 times: see also 'Breathing & Voice 2', below.

1. Breathe in through the nose to a count of 4 and out through the mouth to a count of 4; keep the shoulders relaxed and the tummy tucked in. Repeat with a pause for 4 counts between breathing in and out.
2. Take a deep breath in through the nose and breathe out on the word 'home'.
3. Say, 'ho, ho, ho', as loudly as possible; repeat more loudly and repeat more softly.

2 Strong movement

1 Invite the group to scatter around the room and call out 'freeze' –everyone stands absolutely still. Then call out 'go' and everyone moves again. Repeat several times until unison is achieved.

2 Encourage contrasts, such as running around in a circle and scattering all over the place.

3 Move around the room as if being blown.

4 Run around and jump very high.

5 Stand absolutely still and create a silence.

3 Rhythm & drum work

1 Invite the group to sit in a circle and clap a simple rhythm until it is clapped in unison.

2 Divide the group in half, one clapping the first rhythm and the second the same rhythm, but twice as fast.

3 Play with the idea of different rhythms: invite the group to make suggestions.

4 Allow group members to use a drum and lead the rhythm: they lead and the group copies.

5 Use a drumming CD and suggest that everyone copies a rhythm.

4 More rhythm & drum work

1 Using a drumbeat, suggest everyone walks to the beat.

2 Try marching to the drumbeat, first on the spot and then around the room.

3 March with a partner and synchronise your movements.

4 March with three people to create a marching 'wheel': the person in the centre marches on the spot and the other two march around in a circle (quite a challenge!).

5 Attempt to march backwards, still marching in the wheel (a big challenge!).

5 Breathing & voice 2

Exercises to be repeated 3 or 4 times.

1 Breathe in through the nose to a count of 4 and out through the mouth to a count of 4; keep the shoulders relaxed and the tummy tucked in. Repeat with a pause for 4 counts between breathing in and out.

2 Take a deep breath in through the nose, and breathe out on the word 'home'.

3 Say, 'ho, ho, ho' as loudly as possible; repeat more loudly, repeat more softly.

4 Repeat quickly: 'red leather, yellow leather' five times, then ten times.

5 Repeat quickly: 'a clown with a crown' five times, then ten times.

6 Talk a nonsense language with a partner as quickly as possible, and then very slowly, as if feeling sleepy.

6 Physical

1 Throw the soft ball around the room to each other while running; vary by throwing the ball while shouting the name of the person to catch it.

2 Hold hands in a circle and pull each way; keep the circle intact.

3 Hold hands in a circle and move over and under each other's arms until a tight knot is formed. Slowly undo the knot without letting go of the hands.

4 Pass a clap or pass a rhythm to create a ripple effect as if it is continuous.

5 Stand in a circle: each person sits down, one at a time. If two go down at the same time, you have to start from the beginning again. Repeat the exercise, but standing up from sitting.

7 Synchronised games

1 Everyone stands in a large circle: each person takes one step forward, but if two people move at the same time the game starts again.

2 Repeat the exercise by moving out of the circle, one step at a time.

3 Everyone stands in a large circle and counts, '1, 2, 3, 4'. On 4 everyone looks at someone else: if two people are looking at each other, they change places. Keep repeating until there has been plenty of movement across the group.

4 Variation: number everyone in the group (going around the room, each person says their number); call out two numbers and those people have to change places.

5 More difficult: call out two sets of numbers, such as 2 and 7, or 4 and 8. People should take care not to bump into each other when crossing the group.

8 Clapping & rhythm

1 Pass a single clap around the circle, one person following the next in the same rhythm.

2 Repeat in the opposite direction, varying the pace if group is ready.

3 Change to a double clap and send it around in one direction.

4 Vary the pace and send it in the opposite direction.

5 Change to a triple clap and send it in one direction, at the same time sending a double clap in the opposite direction.

9 Chants & rituals

1 Share the idea that certain jobs have their own chants, so that everyone works together, for example: pulling a rope, rowing a boat.

2 Invite everyone to sit in a circle and teach the chant: 'Aayee oh, aayee oh, ay, ay, ay, ay, aayee oh'. Practise until synchronised.

3 Add the movement of rowing a boat to the rhythm; practise until chant and movement are synchronised.

4 Remind the group that words have rhythms and that chants are based on words and sounds. Invite members to think of phrases that others say: 'Its goodnight from him – and goodnight from me'; or 'Nice to see you – to see you nice'.

5 Introduce the theme of words and music having rhythms; invite group members to think of music they like with a strong rhythm and words, and practise it together.

10 Rhyming words & rhythmic words

With a rhyming dictionary

1 Invite the group to sit in a circle and clap, while saying words that rhyme, for example: splat, mat, cat, rat …; or hi, my, try, cry, fry …

2 Share words that have a strong rhythm, such as; dinner, dinner, dinner; or hokey, cokey, cokey, cokey.

3 Invite everyone to make up two lines that rhyme: 'I went to school and broke a rule'; or 'I went to school and fell in a pool'. Encourage more and more nonsense: 'I went to school, riding a mule.'

4 In pairs, write down (or just say) as many words as possible that rhyme with 'song' (the rhyming dictionary lists 21); then add slight pronunciation variations, for example, 'tongue'.

5 Ask people to form pairs and give them a first line, such as, 'Today I am going to cook a song'. Each pair adds three more lines that rhyme.

11 Drama & focus games

1 Varoom: standing in a circle, one person calls 'varoom' and looks at someone else; that person says 'varoom' to another, and so on. You cannot 'varoom' someone next to you, and there should be no repetition back and forth to same person.

2 Varoom Plus: 'varoom' someone in the group, who then chooses to call 'bazooka' and holds both arms out in front of them, hands clasped, pointing towards someone on opposite side of group. Or they call out 'varoom plus', at which everyone crosses their arms on their chest and the leader starts Varoom Plus again.

3 Variation: as above, but a including a third action and sound, 'lalala'. If someone shouts 'lalala', everyone else has to put their hands over their ears and shout, 'lalala' four times!

4 Invite members of the group to add an action with a nonsense word, but ask them to avoid movement that could lash out at others: keep all extended movement to the front, rather than to the side.

5 Invite members of the group to choose one of the games to practise very quickly.

12 More drama & focus games

1 Bees Knees: everyone runs around the room with one hand on one knee and calls out 'bees knees'; each person has to touch four pairs of knees, and then repeat, remembering which knees they touched the first time!

2 Aliens: everyone stands in a circle. The leader in the middle turns slowly around and then points with clasped hands towards one person, calling 'Medan'; that person ducks and the people on either side face each other and call out 'Nimro'; the person ducking calls back 'Feelib', and can stand up again. If anyone says the wrong name, then they have to stay on one knee; repeat until everyone is an alien or everyone is out because they made three mistakes (one knee, second knee, then the person sits on floor).

3 Slapping hands: kneel in a circle and place the left hand, palm down, to the front; place the right hand to right of the next person's left hand, so that hands alternate around circle; send a slap around the circle, to the right, from left hand to left hand!

4 Repeat from right hand to right hand, to the right.

5 Try sending the slaps in the opposite direction, moving to the left, (requires patience and skill!)

13 Rhyming & nonsense play

1 'I did not go to school because ...' Everyone thinks of the silliest reason, such as: 'I met a bulldozer on the way', or 'It was raining ice-cream', or 'It was Sunday anyway.'

2 'We cannot play football because ...' 'They have planted potatoes on the pitch', or 'The guinea pig ate the football', or 'They are playing hockey instead.'

3 In pairs spaced out around the room, Partner 1 mimes a job and Partner 2 asks, 'What are you doing?'. The response is a nonsense answer. For example, if they are miming digging the garden, Partner 1 might answer 'fixing the bike', or 'mixing a cake', or 'blowing my nose'.

4 As above, but continued. For example, when Partner 1 answers 'blowing my nose', Partner 2 starts to mime blowing their nose.

5 As above, but continued. For example, when Partner 2 is miming blowing their nose, Partner 1 might respond with: 'Why are you going to sleep? I said I was blowing my nose'. And then Partner 1 does something else entirely; for instance they could mime feeding birds.

14 Games for Improvisation

1 Run a three-legged race with a partner without tying the ankles together.

2 Create stepping stones across an imaginary river or chasm with pieces of newspaper. Everyone needs to cross without tearing the paper; elaborate with two people working together and moving onto each piece of paper at the same time.

3 The group pretend they are medical students and someone comes to give them a talk on knitting.

4 The group pretend they are housewives and househusbands, and someone comes to give them a talk on brain surgery.

5 Two people are fruit and vegetable stall holders and call out what they are selling, with the prices; they try to compete with each other.

6 In partners, one person is a customer and the other is trying to show all the best points of a car – but they know nothing of cars, so they have to bluff their way through.

7 In partners, one is a student and the other a physics teacher – but in reality they are a piano teacher and know nothing about physics.

8 In small groups, one person leads the others across different terrain, such as a desert, a rain forest, an ice flow, a stream, a farmyard, and so on. Group members don't know what the terrain is, so they follow and then guess at the end.

9 Repeat, but pretending that the ice is about to crack, or there will shortly be a landslide, so everyone has to move quickly and lightly.

All of these exercises can be developed into situations or stories. Many will become favourites to be repeated. Very importantly, group members will start to develop their own versions of the exercises.

Appendix 2
Recipes

The following recipes have been carefully chosen for working with teenagers who have attachment difficulties. They are simple 'nurture' foods and also encourage healthy eating. When cooking facilities are not available, choose one of the uncooked dishes (see 'Broken Biscuit Cake' or 'Oat Cakes with Nuts, Dates & Raisins'), which provide instant gratification!

Please note: there are many more recipes on the internet that can be added to those listed below and teenagers themselves might like to search online for favourite recipes that they would like to try. It is important to find a compromise between instant food and food that takes too long to prepare in your setting.

NB Always be alert to food allergies.

Nurturing Drinks

For teenagers who are used to buying a sugary, fizzy drink for breakfast, the introduction of different drinks may take time. However, persevere and see whether they are willing to experiment.

Nurturing hot drinks

Hot chocolate, or hot milk and honey (for example) are particularly nurturing. Try to use cocoa and add milk and a small amount of sugar or honey, rather than ready-made chocolate powder.

Home-made lemonade

Ingredients 2 unwaxed lemons
2 oz (57 g) citric acid
1 lb (454 g) sugar
2 pints (1130 mls) boiling water

Required Grater to remove lemon zest, sharp kitchen knife, wooden spoon, earthenware jug or bowl

Method Wash the lemons and grate a small amount of zest into the jug/bowl. Cut the lemons in half; squeeze and add their juice, pips and skin to the jug/bowl. Add sugar and slowly stir in boiling water, making sure all the sugar dissolves.

Leave to stand until cool, then fish out the lemon halves and pips (or use a strainer, although this takes out all the lemon zest). This is a very concentrated lemonade: use only a small amount per glass and dilute it with water.

Nurturing Food

Porridge

Simple porridge can be cooked on a stove or in the microwave. If absolutely necessary, the instant version in pots can be tried!

Ingredients Porridge oats
Sugar, or preferably honey
Raisins (optional)

Required Non-aluminium pan or microwave bowl, wooden spoon, measuring jug

Method Allow 2 parts of water to one of oats. Follow the instructions on the packet, as cooking times vary, but the porridge is ready it in a matter of minutes. The raisins help to sweeten, which means added sugar (or honey) can be kept to a minimum.

Less Sweet Food

Oat cakes with nuts, dates & raisins (uncooked)

Ingredients 2 cups walnuts
1 cup fresh dates, or soak compressed dates
1 cup porridge oats
3 drops vanilla essence
Salt
½ cup raisins
Extra chopped nuts and oats, to finish

Required Food processor, mixing bowl, wooden spoon, greaseproof paper

Method Place the walnuts, then the dates, in a food processor until they are chopped and well mixed; add the other ingredients, except for the raisins, until well blended. Put into a mixing bowl and add the raisins; mix well.

Turn onto greaseproof paper and mix like dough. Divide into small cakes and roll these in chopped nuts and oats.

Broken biscuit cake (uncooked)

If you can save broken biscuits in advance, this recipe will be much cheaper than buying digestive biscuits and then crushing them with a rolling pin inside a plastic bag.

Ingredients 8 oz (250 g) broken digestive biscuits
10 oz (300 g) cooking chocolate
3½ oz (100 g) butter
3 tablespoons runny honey (or golden syrup)
3 tablespoons raisins
chopped nuts (if desired)

Required Rolling pin, mixing bowl, wooden spoon; bowl, saucepan, water and hob to melt chocolate; small, square baking tin, greaseproof paper, access to a refrigerator

Method Pound the biscuits into small pieces and powder with the rolling pin, then put in a mixing bowl. Melt the chocolate with the honey and butter in a bowl over a saucepan of hot water. Mix the chocolate mixture into the biscuits and add the raisins (and chopped nuts, if desired). Press into a small square tin, lined with greaseproof paper. Divide into squares and place in a fridge to set.

Sweet & Spicy

Sweet potato fries

Sweet potatoes can be used as a more healthy alternative in many regular potato recipes.

Ingredients sweet potatoes
rosemary
olive or coconut oil

Required Scrubber to clean potatoes, knife, baking tray, access to an oven

Method Pre-heat the oven to 180–200°C (350–390°F). Scrub the sweet potatoes and slice them lengthwise into chip portions. Place on a baking tray and sprinkle with rosemary and olive or coconut oil; bake in the oven for 20 minutes. Could then be eaten with a yoghurt and chilli dip.

Sweet potato curry

Ingredients 2 tablespoons of korma curry paste
2 sweet potatoes
14 oz (400 g) tin of coconut milk
14 oz (400 g) tin of pineapple chunks, in water not sweetened juice
Rice as side dish, if desired

Required Knife, saucepan and hob, wooden spoon

Method Peel the sweet potatoes and cut into chunky pieces; heat the korma paste in a saucepan and mix in the sweet potato chunks. Put in the coconut milk, adding a little water if the consistency is too thick; cook for about 15 minutes until the potato is tender, but not mushy; add pineapple, stir well. Serve with rice, or use as a snack dip.

Sensory Food

Baking bread

Ingredients 3 cups bread flour
1 teaspoon sugar or honey
2¾ teaspoons active dry yeast
Large tablespoon coconut oil
1 teaspoon salt
1¼ cups milk
½ cup warm water

Required Mixing bowl and wooden spoon, two small, greased loaf tins, tea towel, access to an oven

Method Put the warm water into a bowl and sprinkle in the yeast; leave to stand until it froths, and then add the milk, honey and oil. Add the flour, mixing well, and allow to stand for a few minutes. On a floured surface, knead the dough well and divide between 2 small loaf tins; the dough should only half fill the tin.

Cover with a tea towel and leave to rise for an hour. Pre-heat the oven to 175°C (350°F). Bake for roughly 30 minutes, until firm when touched.

Banana bread

Ingredients 2–3 ripe bananas (skins should be black, or nearly so)
⅓ cup melted butter
½ of runny honey
1½ cups bread flour
1 large egg (beaten)
1 teaspoon vanilla essence
1 teaspoon baking soda
Pinch salt

Required Mixing bowl, fork and wooden spoon, saucepan to melt butter, access to an oven, 4 × 8 in (10 × 20 cm) greased loaf tin, access to an oven

Method Pre-heat the oven to 175°C (350°F). Mash the peeled bananas with a fork and add the melted butter; mix the baking soda in carefully, then add the salt, followed by beaten egg and vanilla. Stir in the honey (warmed, if necessary, for easier blending). Mix in the flour to make a thick batter. Pour into the loaf tin and bake for 50 minutes or a little more – a sharp knife should come out clean when inserted. Allow to cool.

Easy naan bread

Since it takes 55 minutes, bear this in mind when planning the lesson time. You need enough time to both cook the naan and eat the food!

Ingredients 1½ cups warm water
I tablespoon sugar
2 teaspoons active dry yeast
1 teaspoon salt
3 cups flour, plus a little extra for the baking board

Method Mix the warm water, sugar and yeast in a bowl, allow to stand until foamy (about 5 minutes)

Mix in thoroughly the flour and salt, then kneed well until it forms a ball. Keep in bowel, making sure it is well oiled; cover with wet and wrung out cloth and put in a warm space. It will take up to 45 minutes to rise a little.

Turn on to floured baking board and divide into 8 portions. Roll out to thick (⅛") oval naan shape, and grill on each side for 2 minutes.

Celebratory Food

Pizza for all

Ingredients 2½ cups plain flour
2¾ teaspoons baking powder
1 tsp salt
1 tsp oil
¾ to 1 cup water
Ingredients for toppings (see below)

Required Mixing bowl and wooden spoon, rolling pin, pizza baking tray, access to an oven

Method Pre-heat the oven to 200°C (390°F). Put all of the dry ingredients into the mixing bowl and mix well. Add oil and water, enough to make a stiff but pliant dough. Knead well for several minutes and roll into a circular shape; place it on an oven pizza tray. Add toppings and bake for about 15–20 minutes.

Toppings Tomato paste and grated cheese; pineapple slices; several different vegetables, cheeses and olives; herbs to sprinkle on top.

Flapjacks

Ingredients 7¼ oz (200 g) unsalted butter
7½ oz (200 g) runny honey
3½ oz (100 g) demerara sugar
14 oz (400 g) porridge oats
Tablespoon of dried fruit, nuts or desiccated coconut (optional)

Required Saucepan to melt butter, mixing bowl and wooden spoon, shallow 8 × 12in (20 × 30cm) greased baking tin, access to an oven

Method Pre-heat the oven to 180°C (350°F). Melt the butter in a saucepan and add the sugar and honey (and optional flavourings); make sure the sugar has dissolved, then add the oats and mix thoroughly. Turn into the baking tin and smooth. Bake for 15–20 minutes. The edges should be crisp and the flapjack slightly soft in the centre. Cool in the tin, and then cut into squares.

Broken biscuit cake

The recipe for the 'Broken Biscuit Cake' (see above, under 'Less Sweet Food') can also be used for a celebratory cake. Place the mixture in a shallow cake tin and, when it has set in the refrigerator, decide on decoration and icing.

Sticky rice balls or Zongzi

Ingredients 2 cups of white rice
3 cups of water
½ teaspoon salt.

Required Two or three saucepans for the rice and the fillings, hob, greaseproof paper or rice paper, ingredients for fillings

Method Rinse the rice thoroughly. Put the rice in a saucepan, covered with water, and bring it to boil over medium heat until the water drops below the level of the rice and small holes appear. Cook for a further 15 minutes on a low heat. Shape into a rice balls with a cooked filling inside (see below) and wrap in greaseproof paper or rice paper (traditionally bamboo or corn leaves are used).

Fillings Chopped walnuts, mushrooms, beans, eggs, sweet potato, fruit, dates, or several ingredients combined; the ingredients should be cooked in a saucepan.

Although this recipe uses conventional white rice, there is also a 'sweet' or 'glutinous' rice that can be used to make sticky rice.

Appendix 3
Ideas for Messy Play with Teens

1. Tear up newspapers into confetti sized pieces. On a count of 3, throw them in the air to create a snowstorm. Repeat.
2. Use the newspaper confetti to have a snowball fight
3. Mix the newspaper confetti with white glue to create *papier mache* and soak overnight, then mix well.
4. Use mixture to model a small statue or animal or landscape
5. Create a mask by smoothing a thin layer onto a plastic mask and wait to dry solid then paint and varnish with a diluted layer of white glue.
6. Alternative mask can be created by modelling a mask shape, allowing to dry, then painting and varnishing.

Please note: a firmer surface can be obtained by varnishing before painting as well as afterwards.

Eco-Messy Play

1. Jump on all the plastic bottles before re-cycling
2. Take glass jars and bottles to bottle bank and enjoy the smashing sound!
3. Use paper from the shredder to throw and play before it is re-cycled.
4. Use one of the cooking recipes to mix and make in a large quantity and give to local homeless people.

Everything that can make a mess can then be transformed into some kind of form: An art object, some cooking, some rubbish. First make the mess and then transform it!

Appendix 4
References

Ainsworth, M. & Bowlby J., 1969, *Child Care and the Growth of Love*, Pelican, London.

Bomber L.M., 2014, *Inside I'm Hurting*, Worth Reading, London.

Bowlby, J., 1969/1999, *Attachment and Loss*, Volume 1. Basic Books, New York

Brown F., 2008, 'The Fundamentals of Playwork', Brown F. & Taylor C. (eds) *Foundations of Playwork*, Open University, Maidenhead.

Bruner J.S., Jolly A. & Sylva S. (eds), 1976, *Play: its role in development and evolution*, Penguin, London.

Erikson E.,1965/1995, *Childhood and Society*, Vintage, London.

Gross M., Stephens G.J., Silbert L.J. & Hassan U., 2010, 'Speaker-listener neural coupling underlies successful communication', *Proceedings of National Academy of Sciences*, Princeton University Press, Princeton, NJ, pp 14425-14430.

Hunter K., 2014, *Shakespeare's Heartbeat: Drama games for children with autism*, Routledge, Hove.

Jacobs A., 2013, *Supporting Teenagers Through Grief and Loss*, Hinton House, Buckingham.

Jennings S., 2015, *101 Ideas for Focus & Motivation*, Hinton House, Buckingham.

Jennings S., 2014, *101 Ideas for Positive Thoughts & Feelings*, Hinton House, Buckingham.

Jennings S., 2013, *101 Activities for Social & Emotional Resilience*, Hinton House, Buckingham.

Jennings S., 2013, *101 Ideas for Managing Challenging Behaviour*, Hinton House, Buckingham.

Jennings S., 2011, *Healthy Attachments and Neuro-Dramatic-Play*, Jessica Kingsley, London.

Jennings S., 1999, *Introduction to Developmental Play Therapy*, Jessica Kingsley, London.

Jennings S., 1998, *Introduction to Dramatherapy: Ariadne's Ball of Thread*, Jessica Kingsley, London.

Jennings S., 1995, *Theatre, Ritual and Transformation: The Senoi Temiars*, Routledge, London.

Jennings S., 1990, *Dramatherapy with Families, Groups and Individuals*, Jessica Kingsley, London.

Lowenstein L. (ed.), 2010, *Assessment and Treatment Activities for Children, Adolescents and Families*, Champion Press, Toronto.

Lowenstein L., 2002, *More Creative Interventions for Troubled Children and Youth*, Champion Press, Toronto.

Maclean, P.D., 1985 'Evolutionary psychiatry and the triune brain', *Psychological Medicine*, 15(2), 219-221. Accessed 4/2/2018.

McFarlane P., 2012, *Creative Drama for Emotional Support: Activities and exercises for use in the classroom*, Jessica Kingsley, London.

McFarlane P., 2005, *Dramatherapy: Developing emotional stability*, David Fulton Publishers Ltd., London.

Miles L., 2010, *Holding On and Hanging In*, BAAF, London.

Miller A., 1997, *Breaking Down the Wall of Silence: To Join the Waiting Child*, Virago, London.

Newham P., 1999, *The Healing Voice*, Vega, London.

Pearson M., 2004, *Emotional Healing and Self Esteem*, Jessica Kingsley, London.

Seligman M., 2011, *Flourish: A New Understanding of Happiness and Well-Being*, Nicholas Brealey, London.

Seligman M., 2002, *Authentic Happiness: Using New Positive Psychology to Realise Your Potential For Lasting Fulfilment*, New York, Free Press.

Souter-Anderson L., 2015, *Making Meaning: Using Clay Therapy with Children and Adolescents*, Hinton House, Buckingham.

Sutton-Smith B., 2001, *The Ambiguity of Play*, First Harvard University Press, Harvard, MA.

Van der Kolk B., 2015, *The Body Keeps the Score*, Penguin, London.

Wolynn M., 2016, *It Didn't Start with You: How Inherited Family Trauma Shapes Who We Are and How to End the Cycle*, Penguin, New York.

Winnicott D., 1974, *Playing and Reality*, Pelican, London.

Shakespeare's Plays

A Midsummer Night's Dream

Romeo and Juliet

Henry V

Twelfth Night

Resources

Teenage Life Blob Cards (Pip Wilson & Ian Long), 2008, Routledge, London.